Hair today...Gone Ha

Foreword - Prof. Romesh Gupta MD,
Introduction - Ravi Bhanot, MRPharmS Dip (Hom.) Dip (Nuu.)

Chapters:

- -

Foreword

The knowledge of trichology (science related to hair) is poorly understood whilst problems related to hair including receding hairline, postmenopausal thinning and other hair disorders remain a major concern to all adults. We know that the psychological impact of losing ones hair can be enormous as this can be seen as a symptom of lost youth or looking unattractive whereas healthy hair and scalp gives confidence.

I am glad that Ravi Bhanot, Research Pharmacist and Alternative Health Practitioner and also co-founder of The Ayurveda Institute of Europe, has researched centuries old theories as well as new western research in bringing a new holistic approach to keeping our hair for longer. There is increasing evidence that complementary and alternative medicine play an important role in the management of many conditions and its use has remarkably increased in the UK over the last 20 years. This use is likely to increase further if therapies are made available on the NHS.

The publication by Ravi Bhanot "Hair today... Gone Hair tomorrow!" is timely and supports the concept of integrated medicine. The integrated medicine focuses on the whole person including lifestyle and diet and looks after the mental, emotional and spiritual health along with treating the physical symptoms.

This exclusive piece of work not only provides in-depth knowledge about hair and the loss of it but also provides a unique approach to keeping hair healthy for longer by applying both ayurvedic and western science along with dietary advice and Nutrigro® hair products.

I am confident that readers will find this book extremely useful. I wish Ravi Bhanot all the best and enjoyable reading to all the readers.

Professor Romesh Gupta MD, FRCP, FRCP (E), MBA
Professor of Ethnicity and Health, University of Bolton,
Consultant Physician and Governor, Lancashire Teaching Hospitals NHS Foundation Trust

• The Beginning

What causes hair loss or hair thinning? Have we moved on from the time of the Greek physician Hippocrates in figuring out what causes hair loss or hair thinning? Traditional methods and medical research have shown different ways of treating alopecia or hair loss. What one can deduce is that every individual is different and everyone's individual circumstances need to be considered to assess the best course of action.

This book has been written after 15 years of research stretching four continents and visiting people of different cultures, backgrounds and colours. *Well you have to have an excuse for travelling!*

I have written this book taking into account what I have seen that works and looking at the many studies that have been carried out on hair loss over the years. This book will give valuable information on scientific, dietary and life style ways to improve hair rather than information on hair transplants or hair pieces. It gives the **nutrition for hair growth - Nutri(tion) for gro(wth)** - *Nutrigro®*. If it has not helped in any way to keep your hair healthier or for longer please email me ravi@coolherbals.com and I will return your money back to you If it has helped, let me know and I will gladly publish your success story for you.

People with thinning hair or those losing hair will find this book helpful in being informed of the various ways forward for them - in an informative, easy to read and understand manner. The objective is not to make you an expert in this topic but to give you enough informed knowledge for you to make a decision that would be best for you. If you are a sucker for more knowledge or want more personal help online email me at ravi@coolherbals.com.

There are an estimated 60 million people in Europe and about the same number in the United States who suffer from some form of hair loss *(I guess you must be one of them otherwise why would you be reading this - unless like me you too have some sort of passion in this topic).*

By the age of 50 over 50% of men and around 25% of women have experienced some form of hair loss (at least we men win in something). This is usually seen as a receding hairline in the front part of the head (temporal) or baldness or hair thinning in the crown area.

Hair today...Gone Hair tomorrow! People are conscious of hair loss and its effect on the image of themselves. *Don't believe me? go and see the hair shelves in supermarkets and pharmacies!* Is it therefore not surprising, that this industry is worth around £4 billion in Europe and the same in the United States? Is this figure set to increase? You bet! - Unless more read this book and follow plans like the Nutrigro® plan! Pass the message on.

Please read through each part of the book, understand it and see the most appropriate way forward for yourself. Alternatively read the summaries or bold typed wording throughout the Chapters. The *Nutrigro®* Hair Plan that I have devised has been made from the knowledge available to date- from ancient Ayurvedic times to modern research. What I do promise is that by following the advice given you can give yourself every chance to keep your hair for longer!

Ravi Bhanot

MRPharmS Dip (Hom.) Dip (Nutr.) JP

Director, Ayurveda Institute of Europe

"I have written this book taking into account what I have seen that works"

Acknowledgment

"I promise you that by following the advice in this book you can give yourself every chance to keep your hair for longer!"

This book could not have been written without the support of my wife and colleague in our Clinic, Sushma Bhanot, to my PA-Karen Wray who spent many an hour proof reading and having to read my jokes time and time again and my three children Pranav, Varun and Ravina and my niece Vanita for their valuable contribution.

I thank the Ayurvedic physicians who thousands of years ago who came up with the theory of Ayurveda related to hair loss and hair thinning and to modern scientists such as Dr. Robert Young and Dr.M.Mortimer for taking the lead into their research into degenerative illnesses. My special thanks go to my present day gurus- Shri Shri Ravi Shankar, Anthony Robbins, Shri Ram Dev and my parents, B.N and Krishna Bhanot. These teachers have shown me how to get the best out of others- and myself in health and beauty from outside and from within!

"My hats off to them - I can – I am 46, I follow the Nutrigro®️ hair plan and I have a full head of hair to show for it!"

Chapter 1

All you need to know about hair –almost

> *"Before you know about your future see your past – before improving your future hair see what has been and is the state of your hair now"© Ravi Bhanot*

- **Typically we shed between 30 and 100 hairs daily** so we are all losing hair daily. Usually however this hair is replaced.

Before understanding how to slow down hair thinning or hair regrowth, we need to understand what hair is, how it grows and conditions that may play a part in this growth.

- **An average head carries 100,000 - 150,000 hairs.**

 If you don't believe me count them yourself!

- There are a variety of colours in hair - black is the most prevalent particularly amongst the Middle Eastern and Asian countries. In the west we have blondes, brunettes and redheads- only 2% are blondes and red heads. These have a low level of the dark pigment eumelanin and a higher level of the pigment phaeomelanin. Brown hair contains high levels of the dark eumelanin and lower levels of the pale pigment phaeomelanin.

- **Hair's primary function is to regulate temperature.** Human beings being warm blooded animals need to keep their body temperature stable. In cold temperatures muscles attached to the hair follicles contract causing the hair to stand up. This results in warm air being trapped between the hair. Since we have other means to keep warm e.g. clothes, our partners (they can certainly get you heated up), exercise and eating hot curries - the main purpose of hair is cosmetic.

How does hair form?

Hair is made from strong strands of a protein called keratin. Chemically this means oxygen, nitrogen, sulphur, carbon and hydrogen (2). Hair is made up of two types of Keratin - type 1 and type 11. Type 1 is acidic in nature whilst type 11 is basic. Together they make the keratin to form hair and nails. (No wonder many people with alopecia also have problems with their nails- and you thought it was nerves!). The proportions of the individual elements that make up hair differ between people of different ages, sex, type and even in the colour of the hair. Hair is not living. It has no nerves and is difficult to destroy.

 So why have some people's hair been destroyed prematurely?

- **Hair grows in our scalps from follicles**. These are unevenly spread in the scalp - usually in groups of two to five. Each follicle has its own life cycle. It produces about six inches (15cm) of hair annually for about four years. It then falls out and after a short period the whole cycle starts again. *Just imagine if this did not happen you could have used the same hair dye once in your lifetime - no such luck I am afraid!*

Natural hair loss is not a disease.

 When hair loss is excessive or when the pattern of loss is abnormal, we get worried. We lose self-esteem and confidence. Why?

This is the physiology of hair growth

- The base of the tip of the hair in the scalp has a small outgrowth of the skin that looks like a doorknob. This is called the papilla. The papilla contains blood vessels. These supply food to the hair.

- During the growth period the new cell grows and pushes out the older part of the hair away from the papilla. It does so until the hair falls out. *A bad hair day for the old hair you could say!* The pattern of cell growth in this papilla determines the characteristics of the hair - whether it will grow straight, wavy or curly.

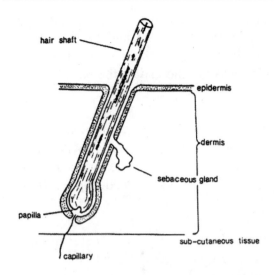

Structure of Hair

- **In adolescence the hair grows at its fastest rate and this reduces with age**

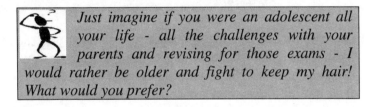

Just imagine if you were an adolescent all your life - all the challenges with your parents and revising for those exams - I would rather be older and fight to keep my hair! What would you prefer?

The cell growth pattern can change due to drugs, pregnancy, illness etc. With age the growth phase of the hair cycle reduces in length and the subcutaneous (below skin surface) of the scalp also becomes thin and the hair becomes more brittle.

Each hair may look like a single fibre but it is made up of three distinct layers- **the cuticle, the cortex and the medulla.**

- The **cuticle** is the layer on the outside. It protects the inner cortex layer. The cells here are flat, hard and horny shaped. Frequently using harsh chemicals on the hair damages the cuticle. When the cuticle breaks at the end of the hair it results in split ends.

- The second layer is the **cortex**. The make up of the cortex determines the strength, elasticity, direction and growth pattern of hair. The width and texture of hair is also determined by the composition of the cortex. The cortex is made up of fibres twisted together, a bit like a rope.

- The cortex gives the colour of the hair. There are four natural pigments- black, brown, yellow and red. What determines the colour and shade of hair is:
  1. The amount of pigment and
  2. Amount of air space in the cortex

(Of course your parents' and your genes play a part too!)

- The **medulla** is the inner part of the hair. It is made of soft keratin. It is composed of large cells that give the appearance of looking hollow. The medulla may or may not be present in the hair but this does not affect the hair in any way.

- **Every hair has a life cycle of its own.** Each hair grows from its own individual hair follicle. A follicle will produce new cells for a certain period of time. This period is called the growth phase.

- **When the hair follicle enters the rest phase, the hair shaft breaks**. The existing hair falls out and a new hair takes its place. The length of time that the individual hair is able to grow during the growth phase controls the maximum length of the hair.

 How do we keep the hair in this phase?

- The cells on the arms stop growing every couple of months. That is why hair on the arms stays short. **The hair follicles on your scalp let hair grow for many years**, so the hair can grow very long. Each hair grows on average half inch every month in the Anagen (growth period). In the resting phase 30-150 hairs are shed per day. On average around 85% of hairs are in the growing phase and 14% are in a resting state and 1% in the Transitional stage (1). **If the Anagen hair count is less than 80% of the total, the person has true hair thinning.** The loss of a single or few hair generally goes unnoticed as there are hair around the 'lost' hair that are in the Anogen or growing phase. Each hair is replaced every three to five years.

Hair Cycle

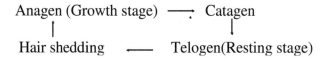

Anagen (Growth stage) ⟶ Catagen

Hair shedding ⟵ Telogen(Resting stage)

- Catagen starts when the Anagen phase comes to an end. **In the Catagen phase cell division stops and the hair stops growing**. The hair follicle shrinks to about one sixth of its normal diameter. Almost 1% of scalp hair is in Catagen phase at any given time. Hair is normally in the Catagen phase for two to four weeks and in the Telogen phase for about two to four months.

> *To understand what is going on the outside we need to know what is going on in the inside. The balance from within keeps the body balance on the outside.*
>
> *This may not be necessarily the conventional western scientists' trail of thought but read on...*

It is said that the body has all the Pharmacy within it. Medicines, food and food supplements help in creating the right environment for the body to repair and renew. The body heals itself. Let us start from the heart.....

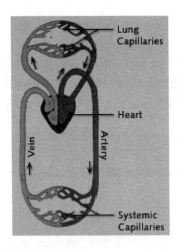

- Blood leaves, the left side of the heart, rich in oxygen. As it passes around the body, blood gives oxygen to these tissues and removes carbon dioxide from them. Blood goes back to the heart through veins and then removes the carbon dioxide through the lungs.

- The lungs exchange the carbon dioxide for oxygen. This then goes through the blood circulatory system to join the left side of the heart. The whole cycle starts again.

- **Poor blood circulation results in not only a poor oxygen/carbon dioxide exchange but also poor removal of toxic waste products from the body.** This results in ill health and acceleration in the ageing process.

- **The areas furthest away from the heart suffer most, particularly fingers, feet and the scalp. A small imbalance in the body affects the hair and scalp.** This could be seen as losing or thinning hair, dry or itchy scalps, dandruff or inflammation. Please bear in mind that the body imbalance could be due to poor circulation, imbalance in hormones, drugs or diet, trauma, stress or due to inherited traits.

Healthy diet and good blood circulation is therefore vital.

The body is more than the elements that make it. The body is holistic and any method that slows down hair loss, hair thinning and reverses hair loss has to take this into account.

Well done you have just learnt the hair cycle!

Chapter 2

Male hair loss - which one is yours?

 "Don't worry about it - we all have to grow old one day - but now is not the time!"© Ravi Bhanot

There are many types of hair loss or alopecia and they affect men, women and children. **Male baldness is by far the most common with over 90% cases being these.** The problem has become more significant in women too. Hair loss can have several causes and underlying reasons.

The types of baldness/ hair thinning or hair loss are: (*identify yours*)

1. **Male Pattern Baldness (Alopecia Androgentica)**
2. **Alopecia Areata- loss of hair in some areas only**
3. **Alopecia Totalis & Universalis**
4. **Traction Alopecia**
5. **Diffuse Alopecia**
6. **Cicatricial Alopecia**
7. **Alopecia Senilis**
8. **Alopecia Adnata**
9. **Alopecia Follicularis**
10. **Alopecia Neurotica**
11. **Trichotillomania**

1. Male Pattern Baldness

> *How to identify: baldness and/or thinning on top of head whilst the sides and back of the head have a strong crop of hair*

The main causes of this type of baldness are: a) genetic: a pattern in the family, b) increased amount of the hormone testosterone being secreted c) age and d) stress.

The stages of hair loss in men MPB.

Typically hair is lost from the temples, the crown and from the frontal hairline.

With further loss the areas of baldness join up to form the common horseshoe pattern.

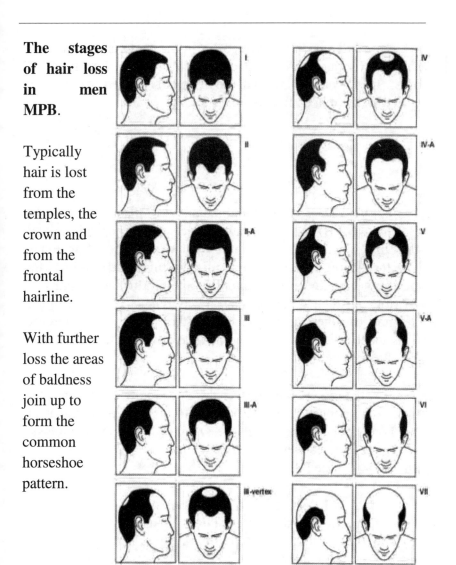

Norwood Classification of Male Pattern Baldness

What causes this pattern of hair loss?

- There have been many theories in the past for this type of hair loss. Strange stories such as **wearing certain tight types of hats; the type of musical instrument played or sexual activities have been** linked to hair loss.

 The mind boggles!

- In 1942 Dr James Hamilton showed that Male Pattern Baldness (MPB) and how much it affects a male depends largely on the interaction of three factors: **Male hormones (Testosterone) or Androgens and how this is affected by the person's genetic pattern and the age of the individual** (1). Aristotle postulated that the reason why Eunuchs (castrated men) did not lose their hair was because they lacked Testosterone. This makes sense as Testosterone is involved in the process of hair loss-see below.

- This theory has been further developed now. Another factor that would appear to play a part is **an enzyme (a chemical in the body that quickens a process) called 5 Alpha Reductase.** This enzyme converts the male hormone Testosterone to Dihydrotesterone (DHT)(2).

- **Increased levels of DHT have been shown to bind to the male hormone receptor sites. These then interfere with the normal functioning of hair follicles.** These hair follicles then cause a gradual, progressive shrinkage in the length and calibre of hair follicles. This process is called miniaturization. Miniaturization results from shortening of the Anagen phase or growth phase of the hair cycle producing progressively finer hairs. 5 - Alpha reductase is found in higher quantities in the scalp of affected people.

- **It is believed that a hair follicle is genetically programmed for a certain number of growth cycles.** The shorter this cycle is in terms of time, the sooner the hair goes through the whole cycle and stops growing new hair. If for example the hair follicle is programmed for fifteen complete growth cycles each lasting an average of five years then the hair follicle will produce new hairs for 75 years (fifteen growth cycles at five years each). **If however the hair follicle is sensitive to DHT in the blood, the growth cycles will shorten from fifteen to complete by the age of fifty or less.** Some hair follicles are programmed to have less than fifteen cycles and this is why you see some men showing a receding hair line before the age of twenty whilst some continue growing hair until the age of thirty or forty.

 Does this make you wonder whether we are similarly programmed before birth?

- **The other effect of DHT on sensitive hair follicles is that it results in thinner and less pigmented hair.** Whereas in normal hair growth, hair grows again after a rest period back to its original same thickness. Hair size in **hair follicles sensitive to DHT do not return to their full size after the rest period**. After each successive growth cycle, the hair follicle reduces in size to an even smaller size. This makes it worse as the affected hair follicles produced by these smaller hair follicles are themselves thinner and less pigmented than normal hair.

- By inhibiting the breakdown of Testosterone to DHT, hair loss can be prevented or at least slowed down.

Testosterone —— DHT—— Hair Loss

- In both males and females with androgenetic or MPB alopecia, the **transition from large, thick, pigmented terminal hairs to thinner, shorter, indeterminate hairs and finally to short, wispy, non-pigmented vellus hairs in the involved areas is gradual,** most would be relieved to know.

- **As hair loss progresses, the Anagen (growth) phase shortens**. As a result, more hairs are in the Telogen (resting) phase. One may notice an increase in hair shedding. The end result can be an area of total baldness.

- This area varies from one individual to another and is usually most marked at the vertex (top of head). **Women with androgenetic hair loss generally lose hair diffusely (thinly) over the crown.** This produces a gradual thinning of the hair rather than an area of marked baldness. The frontal hairline is often preserved in women with this disorder, whereas men note a gradual recession of the frontal hairline early in the process.

- In alopecia that is patterned, an increase in vellus (fine colourless short hair covering most of the body surface hairs) is seen, and fibrous root sheath (fibre looking roots) is seen below reduced sized follicles. **The hair seems patterned as you see long and short hair mixed on the scalp.** In people suffering from long-term hair loss, connective tissue may completely replace hair follicular structures-giving a bald look.

- **Hereditary hair loss happens over a period of time** so dealing with the problem early can sometimes slow the process. In addition, not all hair loss is hereditary. Hair loss may actually have a combination of causes, many of them reversible.

- **Upjohn Pharmaceuticals produced** a tablet to treat high blood pressure called Loniten, which was shown to have a side effect in 80% of patients causing hair growth. They then went on to produce from this the best-selling medicine: **Minoxidil lotion** (brand name Rogaine or Regain) to work solely on the scalp.

- So what does this show us? <u>**It shows us that affecting the chemistry of our blood can play a part in keeping our hair for longer.**</u>

- **In the animal kingdom, baldness is virtually only seen in human beings.**

 (Couldn't be due to our partners could it?)

We can change our diet causing a negative effect to our health and to the growth of our hair more so than any other animal. There are other factors of course that need to be seen to. **Whilst we may not have the control over pollutants and chemical substances in the environment there is however no doubt that blood to the scalp and hair is one major consideration and this is under our control.**

What we can do to keep our blood more revitalized is discussed in the chapter: The *Nutrigro®* Hair Plan.

2. Alopecia Areata

> *How to identify: This is where there is loss in some areas of the scalp*

• **It is seen in males and females** of all ages and races although younger people are more affected. Although this type of hair loss is **seen more on the scalp, it can occur in other parts of the body**. Onset most often begins in childhood. It can be psychologically devastating. It is not life threatening though.

In Alopecia Areata the hair follicles grow so slowly that the hair is not seen above the scalp. **The follicles can grow again with the right nurturing** (3).

What causes this pattern of hair loss?

• This is an **unpredictable, autoimmune skin disease** resulting in the loss of hair on the scalp and possibly elsewhere on the body. The affected hair follicles are mistakenly attacked by a person's own immune system or white blood cells. **This results in the hair growth stage stopping.**

If this condition starts before puberty, the prognosis is not good. Treatment for this condition is not that successful. Topical steroids and topical immunotherapy have been used as has Minoxidil but with limited success.

3. Alopecia Totalis and Universalis

- **Alopecia Totalis is total loss of hair on scalp only whereas Alopecia Universalis is loss of hair throughout the body.** In Totalis this may start as small patches on the scalp and it has now resulted in all the hair on the scalp being lost.

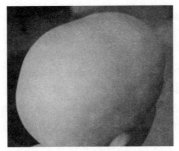 Alopecia Totalis

The hair follicles are below the skin and there is a possibility of the hair growing again. In Universalis, the hair loss goes on throughout the body. **The Totalis and the Universalis are autoimmune diseases** – in other words it is the failure of the body to recognize its own constituent parts. This results in an immune response against its own cells and tissues. Alopecia Universalis is not always disadvantageous.

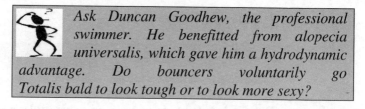

Ask Duncan Goodhew, the professional swimmer. He benefitted from alopecia universalis, which gave him a hydrodynamic advantage. Do bouncers voluntarily go Totalis bald to look tough or to look more sexy?

4. Traction Alopecia

How to identify: receding hairline seen where hair has been pulled

• **Traction alopecia is the hair loss that follows when there is too much tension on the hair. As the hair is pulled it loosens the follicles.** In tight plaiting for example, hair loss is often seen at the frontal hairline and at the sides of the base of the plait.

Is this again for a sexy image?

Devices such as tight ponytails, tight fitting helmets, tightly fitted hair rollers and tight braiding are typical reasons for this type of hair loss. If the hair were under tension for too long it is unlikely that hair would regrow.

5. Diffuse Alopecia

How to identify: diffuse hair loss across whole of scalp

- **Diffuse alopecia is a gradual hair loss everywhere on the whole scalp.** There is no itching or scaling involved. This is seen mostly in women. It may be due to an underactive thyroid, pituitary or adrenal glands or overactive thyroid gland. **Deficiencies in the diet of protein, iron or zinc can cause this type of baldness.**

- **Telogen effluvium is another type of diffuse alopecia. Here the number of hairs lost increases three months after an event.** Some drugs can cause this as a side effect. It is advisable to get medical help in this type of hair loss, as some of the reasons for this hair loss may be serious.

6. Cicatricial Alopecia

How to identify: hair loss is seen in scarred areas only

- This is **hair loss that is seen in areas scarred due to infection, wounds, burns or boils.** In these areas hair follicles don't grow. Hair loss can be diffuse or localized. The causes could be chemical or thermal burns, lupus erythematosus and infections.

7. Alopecia Senilis

How to identify: loss of hair is seen in old people for no apparent reason

This is hair loss due to old age. There is no particular pattern of hair loss. It occurs due to our metabolism slowing down and the normal nutrients, which replenish the follicles not reaching them. As a result new hair does not appear as plentiful as it did in younger age.

8. Alopecia Adnata

- In rare exceptions children are born without hair.

9. Alopecia Follicularis

- Where there is **inflammation on the scalp** hair may not grow at this site.

10. Alopecia Neurotica

- **Hair loss sometimes follows a nervous disorder** or an injury to the nervous system.

11. Trichotillomania

- This occurs where there is **hair loss as a result of pulling your own hair;** sometimes this is done without the person realizing they are doing it. Young children sometimes do this to get the attention of their parents, for example after the birth of a baby in the family.

 Have you figured out your type of hair loss is?

Chapter 3

Hair thinning in women- the top unspoken causes of hair loss-which relate to you?

Hair loss in men can lead to feelings of low self-esteem and feelings of self-consciousness, but the consequences of hair loss in women can be devastating.

The **main differences between male and female baldness** are that:
- **In women, hair loss tends to be over the whole area** of the head and
- **Some on the crown or at the hairline.**
- **Hair loss starts at around 30** and it is more pronounced at around 40.
- **More hair loss is seen at menopause**
- **Hair loss is less common than in men**

Female Pattern type Alopecia

How to identify: thinning hair seen in females with bald areas seen on the scalp

- The hair could be thinning for a period of time-possibly years. **The scalp is seen to be noticeably bald in areas particularly after washing and combing hair.** When the hair dries, the hair appears not to be as sparse.

Ludwig Classification of Female Pattern Baldness

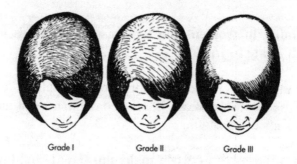

Grade I   Grade II   Grade III

What causes this pattern of hair loss?

• **Stress and hormonal imbalance** may be possible causes for this type of hair loss. Other possible causes affecting the growth of hair may be **some colourants, excessive bleaching or chemicals, some shampoos and hair cosmetics. Some hairstyles or mechanical friction** such as excessive brushing or combing can contribute to this hair loss.

The first step to recovery is to counteract the above possible causes. However if the cause is not dealt with in good time, the hair loss could get worse or the hair loss could be forever.

The causes of hair loss in women can be due to one or more of the following reasons: dietary, genetic, hormonal or psychological. Women who are losing hair need to consider whether any of the following causes are associated to their hair loss:

• **Hereditary.** This is an important factor when it comes to hair loss or hair thinning in both men and women.

- **Low iron count. Iron is needed for hair growth**. A supplement containing iron should remedy the situation. Heavy periods may cause excessive iron loss.

- **Malfunctioning of the thyroid or a hormonal imbalance.** Hormones mediate hair growth and any imbalance could result in follicles going into the resting stage. This would affect hair growth. **Medication to rebalance the thyroid imbalance should help in rectifying the hair loss**. The menopause is another time when hair loss starts.

- **Taking drugs** *(not that sort!)*. A wide variety of medicines cause hair loss or hair thinning as a side effect. Examples are allopurinol, aspirin, carbamazepine, oral contraceptives and warfarin. On no account stop taking these without consulting your doctor. Diabetes, lupus and thyroid disorders have been shown to cause hair loss. **Some cancer treatments cause hair cells to stop dividing making hairs thin** and causing them to break off at the scalp. This occurs up to three weeks after the start of treatment. Patients can lose almost all their scalp hair. The **good news is that hair will regrow** after treatment ends. On balance, it is more important to continue with the drug treatment and accept the hair loss until the treatment is over. It may be possible to lower the dose or to switch to an alternative drug with the same therapeutic effect, but without the hair loss side effect. Speak to your Doctor.

- **Birth control tablets** (oral contraceptives). **Some women who lose hair whilst taking birth control pills usually have an inherited tendency for hair thinning.**
It is the **hormone progesterone that can trigger hair loss in women who are genetically predisposed to thinning hair.** Researchers found that progesterone lowered the level of sex hormone binding globulin (SHBG)(1)-a serum or plasma protein. It was found **that women with a low SHBG were more likely to suffer from more severe premenstrual symptoms. The chances of hair loss are more in women who**

are genetically prone to alopecia areata, who have relatively low levels of SHBG and who are on a progesterone-containing pill.

The hormone Norethisterone is a synthetic form of progesterone. **If you have thinning hair avoid this hormone or Norgestrel-synthetic Norethisterone. Rather than using contraceptive pills such as Norimin, Loestrin 30, Brevinor, TriNovum and BiNovum, which contain forms of oestrogen and progesterone, use pills such as Marvelon, and Dianette.** These contain anti-androgen (male hormones) ingredients. A different form of contraception may be a wiser course of action. Speak to your Doctor about what would be best for you. When a woman stops using oral contraceptives, she may notice that her hair begins shedding two or three months later. This may continue for up to six months when it usually stops. Remember to counteract the effects of progesterone, using a lower dose progesterone pill, or higher oestrogen or an anti-androgen pill.

When a woman is pregnant more hairs are in the growth phase, particularly in the second and third trimester, than in the resting or shedding phases. However, **after childbirth the hair goes back to its regular growth cycles**. Although hair loss can increase in the six months after childbirth, the condition normally rectifies itself.

- **HRT**. There is a fall in the female hormones- oestrogen and progesterone at menopause (a hormone is a chemical that is carried through the endocrine system as a means of regulating or quickening bodily functions). **Oestrogen helps hair growth and thicker hair**. Most Hormone Replacement Therapy (HRT) regimes contain both these hormones. The oestrogen, amongst other things, may help hair growth but the progesterone protects against the possibility of cancer of the endometrium, therefore is necessary in women with a uterus. Women with a hysterectomy are prescribed oestrogen only. It is possible to take an alternative version of HRT. This contains an oestrogen (many are available) plus a natural progestogen, available on prescription as Cyclogest (suppository or cream is available). Another synthetic popular progesterone hormone is Medroxyprogesterone acetate. Medroxyprogesterone acetate is the active ingredient hormone in HRT Tridestra three-month pack. The advantage of this pill is that there is a reduction in number of days one has to take progesterone compared to other HRT medications. **Premique contains oestrogen and medroxyprogesterone and may be more suitable than brands such as Tri Sequens, Elleste, Estracombi, Kliofem and Estrapak.** Hair often comes back after rectifying certain hormonal imbalances.

A Doctor would evaluate a woman's entire medical history individually; assess which HRT medication would be best and would weigh the pros and cons associated with the medication before prescribing it. Women taking any form of HRT should have regular medical gynaecological check-ups and should have their HRT reviewed regularly. Women using HRT also have a slightly increased risk of stroke and blood clots forming in the veins. This risk is higher if there are existing risk factors and needs to be weighed against the personal benefits of taking HRT.

• **Radiation. Exposure to high levels of radiation such as those used for cancer treatment can cause hair loss by affecting the division of cells.** Hair follicles shut down as a result. Hair does normally regrow once the exposure is stopped. However with high doses of radiation there is a risk of hair loss for a long period of time, if not forever.

• **Stress may cause hair to go into the resting phase** and hair loss will increase. Some argue that losing hair is what causes stress in the first instance.

Is high level of stress a cause or a consequence of alopecia or is it both?

There has been an increase in hair loss in women in the past fifty years. Why? **One explanation given by women is that they face an increase in stress and frustration.** The role of women has changed. Where they were primarily housewives looking after the children and home, many now go to work and take on roles that were the domain of men as well as looking after a family, home, elderly parents, no wonder, stress plays a part.

This is not to say that women fifty years ago did not work hard or did not have stress. There may have been more of a united feeling in those days as more women felt they were in the same position. This feeling of understanding in itself helps lessen stress.

It needs to be pointed out that evidence implies that **stress is unlikely to play a major role in causing hair loss, but stressful life events may act as a trigger** in starting and/or making hair loss worse (3). What is the solution to this extra strain? Consider meditation, yoga and just taking the time to breathe more slowly and deeply to reduce stress-see *Nutrigro®* plan. Enjoy today!

Severe ill health and surgery

Fungal infections in the scalp can damage hair follicles. Hair growth can be affected as a result. **Infections, which cause irritation and scratching, can cause mechanical damage to the hair.** There is some evidence, although not conclusive, that a viral infection could cause alopecia. Some have suggested that a **bacterial or viral infection may lead to the immune system being compromised. They then attack the hair follicles in some susceptible people**. It is advisable to use a Shampoo with a natural broad spectrum antibacterial, anti-fungal and anti-viral in it, such as Tea Tree Oil. Try *Nutrigro®* Shampoo.

Hair loss may be due to unbalanced diets, fasting or crash dieting. The possible reasons may be a deficiency in Vitamin C or E, Beta-carotene or other antioxidants. A supplement containing these would be beneficial when one is dieting.

 Ladies: Is it beginning to make more sense yet?

Chapter 4

Bad hair days: Other hair loss causes in males and females-are any yours?

> *"To appreciate the good days one has to appreciate the bad days"© Ravi Bhanot*

It is true to say that we are a long away from fully understanding all the causes of alopecia. There are a number of possible causes. **However we need to understand the causes before we can counteract them.**

1. Toxicity

- **The cause of this type of hair loss is due to chemicals and toxins from the environment, ingestion and by chemicals that we put on our hair via shampoos and conditioners.** Side effects of chemicals are becoming more apparent possibly as their usage and variety has increased. Examples of drugs/ chemicals that may have possible toxic side effects include: formaldehyde (preservative), drug zidovudine (drug used for HIV) and fluvoxamine (an antidepressant).

> *What makes it difficult to prove in fluvoxamine-an antidepressant, is whether the alopecia caused the depression or vice versa.*

This type of hair loss is also seen after certain illnesses such as malaria and typhoid fever. Ingestion of various poisons cause hair loss. The following have been implicated- mercury, warfarin (in large doses), overdose of Vitamin A and boric acid, a common household pesticide, used over a period of time.

2. Psychosomatic-where cause of hair loss is not known

• **Stress and trauma can sometimes cause hair loss**. The type of hair loss is called Telogen Effluvium. This is **characterized by sudden diffuse hair loss** caused by an interruption in the normal hair growth cycle. This is seen in people who worry about their hair or hair loss and this triggers hair loss itself. Some scientists believe that alopecia is an autoimmune disorder. This is where the person's own immune system attacks its own tissue thinking that it is foreign. **Stress is linked to the immune system.**

 Despite this belief do you think anyone knows how stress is related to the immune system?
The answer is No.

Research shows however that chronic stress is linked to a decrease in some immune cells.

The **white blood cells (our defence cells) attack the bulb area of the hair follicle causing temporary hair loss. This is quite often seen in Alopecia areata-**hair loss in one or two small patches. Hair does regrow eventually. The size and duration of having these bald patches increases with each successive episode of this disease. Some people lose all the hair on their scalp – a condition called Alopecia Totalis. In more extreme cases hair is lost all over the body-a condition called Alopecia

Universalis. The hair loss can persist for a long period of time. **There is still hope for hair regrowth as the inflammation occurs in the bulb area and this re-grows with each hair growth cycle.**

• The onset of these bald patches is not life threatening although psychologically, particularly in young people, the effect can be devastating. **Standard alopecia treatments such as steroids and Minoxidil lotion have a limited success.** There are other options such as shaving the whole head off, wigs and hair transplants but they too have their advantages and disadvantages. This same autoimmune attack is seen in conditions such as lupus erythematosus. Follow the *Nutrigro® plan* of action too.

 Do you think for some people it is not the alopecia they are concerned with but the stress or their looks that this may bring?

• Stress is part and parcel of life for a lot of people. For most it is a varying amount at some stages in their life. For others it is a daily occurrence. Since it is widespread and has been on the increase over the last few centuries we need to understand stress, how it affects us and how we can control it.
What complicates matters is that hair loss due to stress is delayed by a few weeks to a few months.
After this period hair loss is sudden. Due to the delay in shedding, the person may have even forgotten the stressful event that triggered this loss. The stressful event could have been a death in the family, marriage, divorce, heart attack or an illness.

Would it therefore be reasonable to assume for hair regrowth and slowing hair thinning, one needs to be able to control stress?

- It is believed that **it is not stress but the ability to deal with stress that makes the difference.** Stress begins from a young age when children are crying out for the attention of their parents or teachers, fighting for marks in school and University and then competing with peers in the job market or keeping up with the neighbours. With the advent of technology such as cable television and Internet we have been driven to be a Consumer driven market where both young and old feel tempted to buy the newest gadget around.

- One could argue that it is envy that is driving this pressure; jealousy, greed and worry are probably playing a part too.

Research is difficult in this area as it is hard to have a proper control group for comparison. Also the same incident for one person may be stressful and for another not so. **The direct link we do have is that perceived stress to an individual has a bearing on physical disorders and immune function of the individual.** Reducing stress may restore hair growth. A severe shock can result in Alopecia Universalis: where all the body hair is lost. This condition is more difficult to reverse.

One in 10 adults across the UK is enduring hair loss or premature baldness due to stress problems. Women are suffering more than men with 74% saying they are stressed compared to 59% of men according to a survey carried out on 3000 people. The generation of women who have been trying to do it all – work, maintain a home and relationship and raise children are the worst hit.12% of women say stress makes their hair fall out compared to just 8% of men. Alopecia areata (random bald patches on the scalp) is often a result of stress.

The secret is of course to **learn how to control stress**. Being aware that you are under this negative influence is the first step in order to control it and your hair!

There are various exercises that help in controlling stress. **Yoga, meditation, exercising or reading are amongst the most popular ways of reducing stress** one has to find the most appropriate to themselves.

In our Clinic we see clients, who are losing hair, complaining of consequential effects of increased stress, loss of confidence and relationship problems. The question is what comes first, the chicken or the egg.

 In a restaurant they would answer "depends what was ordered first"-but life is not a restaurant.

3. Infections in men and women

• **Fungal infections such as ringworm (tinea capitis), kerion and favus on the scalp can cause hair loss** (1). Bacterial infections such as folliculitis, furuncles and carbuncles can cause thinning of hair. A good shampoo containing a natural broad spectrum antifungal and antibacterial such as Tea Tree Oil should help (use *Nutrigro®* Shampoo- see *Nutrigro® plan*).

4. Eczema or asthma related

• **There is some research that implies that if you suffer from either of the above you stand a greater chance of suffering from alopecia.** In the US, one study showed that of those that suffered from asthma or eczema or both, 18% children and 9% adults suffered from alopecia areata (2).

 If you have hair loss do you fit in this category?

5. Thyroid and endocrine gland disorders

• Hair loss can be caused by a disorder of the thyroid (3). This endocrine gland controls the metabolism of the body through the hormone thyroxine. Hair loss could be related to other conditions such as diabetes, heart disease, liver disorder or low iron levels in the blood. These can all be tested for and eliminated as possible causes.

• It is interesting to note that studies show that up to 10% of women have thyroid dysfunctions six to twelve months after having a baby. This could be a reason for hair loss after having a baby. An immediate blood test may be recommended in this instance and suitable medication could be prescribed if necessary.

 Would you agree that men and women are prone to hair thinning and hair loss but not necessarily for the same reasons?

Chapter 5

Bonus know how on hair and scalp troubles

- The **skin is made up of five growth layers**. The lowest layer is the Germinative Layer. In this layer cells divide and move upwards. **It normally takes about a month for these cells to push through the intermediate layers of cells to the surface layer.** On moving upwards they flatten and form the Stratum Corneum. At this stage the cells are dead. As the skin renews from within, the dead cells of the Stratum Corneum flake away. The skin is lost constantly in tiny patches.

When this does not happen in this normal way there are scalp problems.

Dandruff

In dandruff or psoriasis, the migration of cells from the lower layer to the surface layer is at a rate, which is faster than normal. To make things worse **there is an increase in microorganism growth on the scalp**. This makes the irritation worse. Dandruff does not cause hair loss.

- **This is a common scalp problem that affects men and women of all ages.** It is seen in dry and even more so in oily scalps. **Typically white loose scales are seen on the scalp surface. There is normal shedding of skin on the scalp. In dandruff there is just a lot more shedding because there is an increase in cells dividing,** a process called mitosis, in the Stratum Germinativum layer. Also in normal stratum corneum (the outermost surface layer of the skin) there are about 30 layers of well-structured keratinised cells whereas in people suffering from dandruff there are only about 10 poorly formed irregular layers.

- **Rather than taking one month for these cells to migrate to the surface layer in dandruff it takes around one week.** There is an increased amount of shedding. There is no permanent cure to dandruff but it can be controlled.

- **Some dandruff appears to be related to the yeast including malassezia** (previously called Pityrosporum ovale) (1). In a single blind test carried out by Satchell and Co. at The Royal Prince Alfred Hospital, Camperdown, Australia with 126 male and female patients there was a 41% improvement in those patients using a tea tree oil shampoo for mild to moderate dandruff. This is why we use this in my formulation of *Nutrigro®* Hair shampoo. There are other shampoos on the market containing ketoconazole (Nizoral) or zinc pyrithione (Head and Shoulders) that could help. Some Dermatologists recommend alternating daily between different active ingredients to control dandruff. **If you have not had the best results by using one particular shampoo then try alternating between the three-*Nutrigro®*, Nizoral and Head and Shoulders.**

Does it matter in which order you use these?

The answer is No.

Otherwise use preparations, which include salicylic acid, tar, selenium, sulphur, and zinc in rotation. If after a few weeks the dandruff condition is no better then see a dermatologist or trichologist.

• Dr. Joseph Bark, of St. Joseph's Hospital in Lexington, KY suggests that because a **high percentage of dandruff sufferers are male, there may be a hormone connection to dandruff.**

• **Dandruff could also be caused by overactive oil glands, food allergies, stress, excessive perspiration, or harsh shampoos.**

• There is **a common misconception that dandruff is caused by too dry a scalp.** As a result some people avoid washing their hair, as they believe that the shampoo would cause a drying effect. **The chances are that their scalp is not being cleansed enough.** The scale builds up into larger flakes before falling off. Dandruff gets worse when hair is exposed to dust, UV light, harsh chemical based shampoo or hair dyes. These cause an increase in number of microbes. These microbes cause unhealthy residue over the scalp. This leads to dandruff and an unhealthy scalp. Consequentially this results in unhealthy, lifeless hair and may result in excessive loss of hair too.

• It is believed that **dandruff is usually a result of too much oiliness of the skin and scalp rather than dryness.** Cold, dry air often worsens dandruff.

Message: Massage the scalp (see Chapter 8) to increase blood circulation and to ease tension in the increased tight scalp and use the alternating shampoo regime.

Seborrheic Dermatitis

- **Classically this is seen as an oily scalp with redness and scaling.** In more **chronic conditions there may be crusts formed and there may be weeping.**

- It affects around 3% of the population and is more commonly seen in men rather than women and is seen in young babies and adults 30 to 60 years of age. **Seborrheic dermatitis can also affect the skin on other parts of the body,** such as the face and chest, and the creases of the arms, legs and groin.

- **The underlying cause is not known.** The cause may be different in infants and adults. It **may be due to hormones because the disorder often appears in infancy and disappears before puberty. Sometimes the cause is due to a fungus called malassezia.** This organism is normally present on the skin in small numbers. However its numbers increase in some cases resulting in skin problems.

- Seborrheic dermatitis has also been **linked to certain neurological disorders such as Parkinson's disease and epilepsy.** The reason for this relationship is not known.

Psoriasis

• **This is where the skin and scalp have red patches, which may be scaly.** Control rather than cure is the best that can be offered at present for this. **In more severe cases there may be some temporary mild localised hair loss.**

• **The hair loss is usually not permanent.** The hair loss can be caused by the treatments for scalp psoriasis themselves. Vigorous and repeated treatments can weaken, break hairs or cause hair loss.

• Sometimes the scalp gets inflamed as a result of psoriasis and can lead to hair loss. Treatment needs care in this instance.

• Removing scales forcefully can pull hair from its roots. Be gentle.

• **Psoriasis appears to be a genetic condition in some people.** **Certain stimuli however trigger off Psoriasis in these people-** exposure to streptococcal infections in the throat, alcohol, medicines, local irritation or damage to the skin are typical examples.

• **Psoriasis vulgaris (plaque psoriasis) and Psoriasis pustulosa (pustular psoriasis) are the two main types of Psoriasis.** They differ in severity, duration, location on the body and appearance of the lesions.

> *Message: At our Clinic we recommend the use of tar shampoos, phototherapy, or emollients such as petroleum jelly or oils such as Psoria Oil (containing Coconut oil and Wrightoria Tincture) as possible solutions. Other solutions: Heat by way of sunshine slows down the rate of reproduction of skin cells so try having a hair style that avoids the more sensitive areas, if possible. Use the Nutrigro® Plan.*

Pityriasis Amiantacea

• In **Pityriasis amiantacea the scalp is thick**. There are yellow-white scales that densely coat the scalp skin and adhere to the scalp hairs as they exit the scalp. **Quite often only part of the scalp is affected. The scales are overlapping like tiles on a roof or flakes of asbestos, hence the name.**

• **The underlying scalp skin may appear normal, aside from the scale, or may be reddened or scaly**. There is no obvious underlying cause. The condition is seen more with young women. The cause of this complaint is not known, but psychological reasons are a possibility.

• **Some hair loss is common in areas of pityriasis amiantacea, but hair regrowth is seen with treatment**. The hair loss is sometimes aggravated by the difficulty in combing the hair due to the thickness of scale at the base of the hair shafts. If an infection occurs as well then hair loss may be associated with scarring. This can be permanent.

Neuro Dermatitis

- **This is sometimes referred to as a nerve rash.** Redness occurs causing an itch. This causes scratching, which in turn causes redness. **Dermatitis or eczema is usually drier than psoriasis.** The affected area has a boundary, which is thick and leather like. It is thought **excessive salt in our sweat may be playing a part** in making dermatitis worse. In this type of condition it is thought that the nervous system is under stress.

> *Message: Calming of the skin with emollients would help as well as the Nutrigro® Plan.*

Please note that the above are guidelines only. Personal diagnosis and treatment would be required for the individual by a medical practitioner.

Why?

Sometimes diagnosis between the different types of hair problems can be challenging.

Introduction to Chapter 6

 "When there is no plan then there is a plan - to fail"

The *Nutrigro® Plan*

 So how do you know you have got healthy hair?

Some of the characteristics that healthy hair have are:

1. **Thick and dense**   2. **Not too oily or rough**
3. **Capable of setting or styling**   4. **Full-bodied rather than limp, hair growth regular.**

a) It needs to be borne in mind that **"normal" hair is a relative term.** It refers to the natural hair type of the individual- oily, dry or normal.

b) **In oily hair the sebaceous glands secrete excess oil.** The oil moves down the hair shaft causing the scalp and hair to be too oily. This hair gives the impression that it is lanky and coarse.

c) **In dry hair there is insufficient amount of sebum and oil on the hair causing it to dry out at the cellular level.** Sometimes the scalp is seen as flaky or with dandruff as a result of the dryness. The hair looks less elastic and is more liable to break or damage.

d) **Normal hair is healthy looking.** The hair does not have over dry or over oily roots. It is easier to cope with and look after.

The *Nutrigro® Plan* consists of following:

What the A-list stars hair-care regime is-are you using it?

Immediate ways to stimulate your hair growth through
Shampooing

Himalayan secrets to give you healthy hair through
ancient Ayurvedic head massage

How to energize your hair roots through food-using
the Nutrigro® Diet Plan

See yourself with a headful of hair

Exercise to give you healthier hair

How to use the art of breathing for healthier hair– ancient
Sanskrit technique

> *Let us consider the seven steps in more details in the next Chapters. If you understand why you are taking the relevant steps there is more of a chance that the Nutrigro® plan would be followed and your hair would be given every chance to be with you healthier and longer.*

Chapter 6

Make sure your Hair Care Regime is like cash-dependable." © Ravi Bhanot

What the A-list stars hair-care regime is- are you using it?

The answer is of course only the best. But what is the best? Looking at Supermarket, Pharmacy or Hairdresser shelves there are a whole array of hair care products. Use products that are natural, without harsh chemicals and products that are effective – don't just go for well-known brands!

The Nutrigro® Care Regime

• We accept that due to **some causes such as hereditary, we inevitably cannot stop hair loss but is there something we can do to slow the process of losing hair or it going thinner with hair care products we use?** Any plan has to be holistic-in other words take the whole body into account.

Is it any wonder that most medicated drugs for hair regrowth have limited use?

The body needs the right food. The foods have to be broken down more efficiently, the body needs to be in a healthy state and the condition of the scalp and hair has to be improved. It is then that the body would function in combination with all its parts to work efficiently to keep the hair that we have.

* Lets start with Shampoos and Conditioners.

> *Why does a shampoo work better than water?*
>
> *A shampoo is a surfactant - each of its molecules has a water loving head and an oil loving tail.* ·

The tail of each shampoo molecule attracts oil, grease and dirt whereas the head attracts water but not dirt. **Water molecules on their own cannot clean the dirt or oil from the cuticle.** The water beads up and bounces off when you wash hair with just water.

> *Why does shampoo work better than soap? Soap is made from organic sources like palm oil or human fat mixed with an alkali. Shampoos are synthetically made from petrochemicals.*
>
> *Soap and shampoo are both detergents-they decrease the surface tension of water allowing them to mix in with the natural oil sebum (produced by the follicles' sebaceous glands), as well as with dirt. Soap does however react with metal ions in hard water to form "scum,"-usually a calcium or magnesium salt. This is difficult to remove from the hair. Shampoo however does not react with hard water and so does not leave scum in the hair.*

A lot of synthetic detergents in shampoo do not foam too well on their own, so manufacturers add lather builders such as cocamide MEA or cocamidopropyl betaine.

Many chemical treatments for hair such as shampoos,conditioners, dyes, tints, bleaches, straighteners can weaken hair if used improperly or too frequently. Prolonged exposure also has this effect. The good news is that stopping the treatment and llowing the damaged hair to grow out can reverse the effects of these products.

Shampoos and Conditioners

 Shampoos are used regularly, but what is the effect of shampoos on our hair and scalp?

Shampoos have their main uses:
-To cleanse the hair and scalp
-Remove dirt and sebum
-Remove any styling preparations

 Are all shampoos the same?

No they are not. Some are alkaline based and some are acidic

The acid base range is from 0 to 14 where 7 is neutral and below this number is acidic and above this number is alkaline. Whereas the skin has a pH (parts of hydrogen) of 4.2 to 6.5 the **hair and nails have a pH of 4.5 to 5.5.**

Alkalis and acids have different effects on the hair. **An alkaline shampoo makes the hair cuticle cells swell and lift, leaving the hair with a rough, dull texture.** An acidic shampoo will seal moisture leaving the hair smooth and shiny.

Bleaches, hair colours, permanents and relaxers are all alkaline solutions made to lift the hair's cuticle to create the desired results.

- **There is <u>no legal requirement to put the pH of a shampoo on a label.</u>** This makes it more difficult for the consumer to know what the pH of their shampoo is.

- **Should the number of times you wash your hair with a shampoo depend on the type of hair you have? Yes is the answer.** If your hair is normal or oily you would need to wash it more often than if you have dry hair. It is a question of balance. If you over shampoo, your hair can look like it is too flyaway and if you do not shampoo enough, the hair can look oily (particularly if you have greasy hair) or not kept well.

- If you do see your hair a little oily there is no need to be concerned.

- **Hair needs a balance between sebum, protein, moisture and acid balance.**

- **Sebum is the natural oil** produced by the Sebaceous gland. This is of benefit to healthy hair as it **protects the hair and skin keeps moisture in the hair, acts as a moisturiser and helps keep friction between hairs to a minimum.**

Protein is essential to making hair.

How much of hair is protein?

97% of hair is keratin, a protein.

This gives the strength and good health to hair. When hair is damaged it is essentially keratin that is damaged.

- **Moisture to the hair gives its elasticity and makes it manageable.** The content of moisture in hair varies between 3 and 14%, depending on the external atmosphere and the amount of relative humidity of water in the air. The moisture acts as a lubricant to the hair.

- **Our skin and hair live in an environment of pH 4.5 to 5.5.** This is the acid level that is produced as a result of the mixing up of sweat and sebum on the skin. **At this pH our hair is in the best environment** to be as strong and flexible as it can be.

A good shampoo needs to be:

Able to form lather
Not to be too concentrated to avoid waste
The pH of the shampoo needs to be between 4.5 and 5.5
needs to be free of harsh chemicals such as Sodium Lauryl Sulphate (or relative of) base shampoo
Natural based
Biodegradable
Not tested on animals

- The effects of air pollution, bathing water and harsh hair care chemicals, emotional or hormonal imbalances have an adverse effect on our hair. They cause the hair to become dry or oily, have split ends or become frizzy. Shampoos can strip away more of your hair's natural sebum. Hair Conditioners were developed to replace hair's natural oils.

- Conditioners are used after shampoos to improve the texture of the hair and to make it more manageable. Its function is to close the cuticle and retain sebum, moisture, acid and protein. Hair is about 97% keratin. Keratin has on its surface amino acids which are negatively-charged. Hair conditioners therefore often contain cationic (positive charged) surfactants. These do not wash out completely, because their hydrophilic (water loving) ends strongly bind to keratin. The hydrophobic (water repelling) ends of the surfactant molecules then act as the new hair surface.

- **Conditioners are moisturisers in some cases**. They are composed of various oils and lubricants. They also contain antistatic components and preservatives for better function in hard water (water with a high mineral content).

- **Conditioners are ideally acidic**. Low pH provides the hair with a positive charge. This allows better forming of hydrogen bonds between the keratin scales. This gives hair more compact structure.

The functions of conditioners are:

1. **Retain moisture and enhances the texture and appearance of hair**
2. **Keep the pH of the hair between 4.5 and 5.5**
3. **Conditioners contain keratin. This protein makes hair fibres strong and fuller**
4. **They are anti-static. They reduce hair going frizzy or being flyaway.**
5. **They protect the hair**
6. **They give back the natural oil that shampoos may have taken away**
7. **They work on the Sebaceous gland so they do not make an excess of oil**
8. **They help keep hair manageable**

There are several types of hair conditioners. They have different compositions and main functions:

Moisturisers. They hold moisture in the hair. Usually contain higher proportion of humectants(absorb water from the air so give moisture to the hair).

Reconstructors. These ususally contain proteins.Their role is to penetrate the hair and strengthen its structure.

Acidifiers keep the conditioner's pH about 2.5–3.5. In contact with an acidic environment the hair's scaly surface tighten up. (The hydrogen bonds between the keratin molecules get stronger.)

Detanglers modifying the hair surface.

Thermal protectors usually absorb heat. They protect the hair against excessive heat caused by blow-drying, curling tongs or hot rollers.

Glossers are light-reflecting chemicals that bind to the hair surface. They are usually polymers, usually silicones such as dimethicone or cyclomethicone.

Oils (E.F.A.'s - essential fatty acids). If you have dry hair, adding oil to your hair can help. The scalp produces a natural oil called sebum. EFA's are the closest substance to natural sebum. Sebum contains EFA'S. EFA's can help make dry hair softer and more pliable.

Conditioners can be described as pack or as leave-in types.

Pack conditioners are heavy, thick and have a high content of surfactants. These are able to bind to the hair structure and cement the hair surface scales together. They are usually applied to the hair for a longer period of time. They tend to form thicker layers on the hair surface.

Leave-in conditioners are thinner and contain different surfactants. They add only a little volume to the hair. They give a lighter, thinner layer on the hair. The difference between leave-in and pack conditioners is almost like the difference between fats and oils.

Ordinary conditioners are usually a combination of both the pack and leave-in ones.

Hold conditioners hold the hair in a desired shape. They are a bit like hair gels.

 So what should a Conditioner for Thinning hair contain?

Conditioners should be natural based, biodegradable with some agent to help give the appearance of thicker hair.

The ideal Formulations of Shampoos and Conditioners

The formulation I recommend and use for hair that is thinning is in *Nutrigro®* Conditioner. It contains a natural emollient and hair building substances, an anti-fungal and bactericidal with our *Nutrigro®* **complex** - an herbal mixture to strengthen hair.

The shampoo formulation I have made for thinning hair is *Nutrigro®* Shampoo. It contains a non-Sodium Lauryl Sulphate SLS base, a palm tree derivative as a foaming agent, an antiseptic (for seborrhoea- accumulation on the skin of the normal sebaceous secretion mixed with dirt forming scales), along with **Tea Tree Oil** (antibacterial and antifungal), **Panthenol** (Vitamin B5-moisturizes), *Nutrigro®* **complex** (containing a herbal extract including Fenugreek herbal extract to strengthen hair **-Phytokeratin** (moisturises and a hair building block), **Saw Palmetto** (slows hair loss),) and Vitamin E) in base.

> *You want the shampoo to be acidic to match the acidic environment of the scalp and hair.*

- **Perspiration and sebum both add to the acidic surface of the scalp of pH 4.5-5.5. At pH 4.5 to 5.5 the hair is at its strongest and least vulnerable to damage and loss of moisture.** This pH also keeps the skin protected from bacterial attacks. Hair that is under the influence of the right pH shines more as the smooth cuticle surfaces reflect rather than absorb light.

To fortify the shampoo I put in other ingredients:

- **Panthenol is a pro-vitamin that penetrates the hair slowly. It improves and moisturises the skin and soothes irritated skin. Research by Roche suggests that hair can be thickened by up to 10% with Panthenol. Panthenol also improves the manageability and shine to hair.** It moisturises the hair shaft to make it appear thicker. It also reduces split ends.

Panthenol causes the hair not to be heavy. It gives a longer lasting hairstyle.

- **Phytokeratin. Keratin is a protein that makes hair. Using keratin in hair and skin gives the basic building blocks to rebuild and condition hair.** Phytokeratin gives all the benefits of keratin amino acids but it comes from a plant source.

- **Phytokeratin is made from a blend of free amino acids. These are in the same proportions as they are found in the human hair amino acids.** Phytokeratin binds the free amino acids naturally present in the sebum and in the hair and in this way keeps the hair moist, supple, strong and acts as a conditioner. Phytokeratin is helped by its low molecular weight as this helps it to penetrate into the hair improving its healthy appearance and adding moisture. Phytokeratin has the advantage over other commonly used proteins in that it will not coat hair in the same way. It gives the hair shine, sparkle and bounce.

- Tea Tree Oil. Sometimes hair loss can be associated with scarring of the scalp tissue due to inflammation and tissue destruction. **Hair loss, as a result of scarring, can occur from infections, either bacterial or fungal.** The hair follicle itself can be blocked, creating further problems such as hair thinning and loss. Tea tree oil has been shown to unblock clogged hair follicles, moisturise the hair and keep the scalp free of bacteria and fungal problems (1).

- Fenugreek has been traditionally used in India, for strengthening hair. In the west it was introduced for bronchitis and as a side effect it was seen to improve hair loss and bring re-growth in some places too. Fenugreek is believed to work by increasing the blood flow to the scalp. The improved blood circulation improves nutrient supply to the scalp.

- **Dry hair requires a gentle, non-detergent based product**; a solution of tea tree oil in a moisturising shampoo may help to unblock sebaceous glands and encourage the flow of the body's own moisturising oils, while clearing away unsightly dead skin cells.

- Ultimately you want a deep cleansing shampoo that cleanses and is nutrient rich for healthy hair growth. **The shampoo should effectively remove build up of sweat, oils, and dirt etc as well as neutralise DHT (Dihydrotestosterone).**

- Research shows that there are herbs that slow hair loss or hair thinning. Some of them work on slowing the conversion of Testosterone to DHT - the process that precedes hair loss.

- Herbs in this class stop the action of the enzyme 5- alpha reductase. This limits the conversion of testosterone to DHT. Finasteride (Propecia) was the first clinically trialled drug to work like this (2). Finasteride has selective activity against 5- alpha reductase. As a result, serum and follicular DHT levels are significantly reduced.

- **Saw Palmetto**. Studies have shown that the herb Saw Palmetto is an effective plant anti-androgen, **in another words it stops the conversion of testosterone to DHT**. It acts in a similar way that Finasteride does (3).

- Firstly **it lowers levels of DHT in the body by blocking 5-alpha-reductase. Secondly Saw Palmetto blocks receptor sites on cell membranes required for cells to absorb DHT.** Although no studies have been carried out on Saw Palmetto and its relation to hair growth, studies have been performed on the use of Saw Palmetto in the treatment of benign prostatic disease. DHT plays a similar part in androgenetic alopecia. Studies that have been performed to date suggest that Saw Palmetto is an effective anti-androgen.

Testosterone $-X \rightarrow$ DHT $\rightarrow$ Hair Loss
        Saw Palmetto slows this reaction

- **Normal healthy hair grows about ½ inch (1.25cm) per month. It takes several months before any effects are noticed.**

- If you are losing hair at the onset of menopause, you can maintain hormonal balance (and consequently hair thickness) with plant-based herbs containing estrogen-like substances so that they mimic the oestrogen ein the body such as soy extract, dong quai (Angelica sinensis) or ashwaganda (Withania somnifera). Other herbs that exert mild estrogenic effects include damiana (Turnera diffusa), black cohosh (Cimicifuga racemosa) and sage (Salvia officinalis). There is not enough evidence for these working in Shampoos to date as yet. The shampoo detergent or cleanser needs to be carefully chosen.

What makes Nutrigro® Shampoo and Conditioner unique?

The Nutrigro® Complex with its enriching herbs and base cleanser make the difference. Using an alternative natural cleansing agent instead of using common agents such as Sodium Lauryl Sulphate or one of its derivatives as the cleansing agent.

Sodium Lauryl Sulphate (SLS) info

Sodium Lauryl Sulphate, Ammonium Lauryl Sulphate and Cocamide DEA are cosmetic detergents. There are many derivatives or relatives to these (Sodium Laureth Sulphate, Ammonium Laureth Sulphate for example). Both have an emulsifying action and thereby **remove oil and soil from the hair and skin.**

In acute eye tests, 10% Sodium Lauryl Sulphate caused damage to the cornea of rabbits' eyes and a product with solutions from 0.1% to 10% has caused skin irritation (4). It should be emphasised that it is safe to use in the common concentrations seen in shampoos- however **minimum hair and scalp contact may be advisable.** Bases containing Castile (made from Olive Oil) and Decyl Polyglucose (derived from corn) or Cocamidopropyl Betaine (derived from coconut oil obtained from the kernels of palm trees) or alkyl polyglucosides (made from a blend of wheat and coconut fatty acids) are milder and less abrahesive alternatives. Cleansing agents such as soapwort (Saponaria Officinalis), soapbark (Quillaja Saponaria), and soapberry (Sapindus Indica) are also suitable. These ingredients will cleanse your hair without swelling the cuticle and causing damage.

· Hair Serums

- Why are natural oils important to hair? **Sebum, our natural oil, keeps moisture in the hair and reduces friction**. Moisture is required to keep hair manageable and give its elasticity. Sebum quantity depends on factors such as hereditary, age, diet, hormones, stress, hair diameter and porosity.

- **Applying a hair preparation for a longer period of time helps sustained effects.** Hair is non-living but **the portion of the hair that lives below the scalp, in the follicle, has frantic cellular activity and life. This leads to the possibility that treatments applied on the scalp that penetrate the oily sebum layers of the follicle should be able to help the growing hair. So the secret to thicker younger hair is to improve follicular health**. Studies have also shown that there needs to be a good capillary (blood) circulation around the follicles to encourage protective nutrients to reach the follicle.

- Traditionally these preparations have been in the form of oils Although this is acceptable in a number of countries particularly in the East, having greasy hair is not socially acceptable in the West.

- **A serum trial with *Nutrigro®* base herbal ingredients** containing a peptide, sugar beet Betaine, fruit extracts, Visnaga Vera (a plant) **amongst other ingredients was conducted to see the effect on hair thickness and hair growth.**

- **The serum appeared to be able to bind to the Androgen Receptor very much like Testosterone. It has also been shown to increase the skin's matrix proteins such as collagen and elastin. This would consequently help improve the scalp and follicles.**

- **The Sugar beet Betaine is believed to improve the production of collagen making the hair bulb stronger.** Betaine also increases production of energy molecules. The extra energy helps the hair function better during the Anagen (growth) phase of the hair.

- **The Fruit extracts in the Serum clear dead cells around the follicles allow thicker hair growth.** The acidic nature of the acids gives the natural pH of the scalp. This would be **perfect environment to keep the hair proteins rigid and breakage resistant.**

- **A molecule called Visnadine present in the herb Visnaga Vera (Umbelliferae family) can help in slightly increasing skin temperature. Increasing microcirculation to the hair roots gives the best conditions for healthy hair growth as it allows oxygen and nutrient delivery to the root of the hair. This improves damaged and weakened hair.**

Chemical structure of Visnadine

C09316

- **A half-head study was used to see if this serum helped hair follicles.** A subjective evaluation of the hair was carried out after using the serum for five days and a scanning electron micrograph was used to compare hair removed from the head that had serum applied to it and that had no serum applied to it.

- **87% of participants felt that their hair was softer and stronger than before the treatment and 66% felt that their hair was smoother after treatment.** The Scanning Electron Microscopy (SEM) showed a significant difference. Pictures show:

Hair follicle after use with control

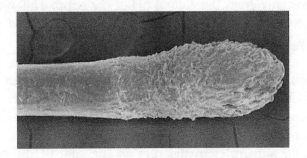

Typical hair follicle removed after use of Nutrigro® Serum base

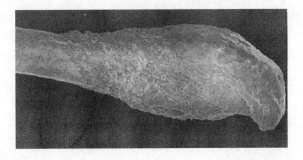

Chapter 7

Nutrigro® Plan - **Immediate ways to stimulate hair growth through shampooing.**

 "Pilots say a one degree change in course can drastically change where you end up - change your shampooing routine a little and see the difference" © *Ravi Bhanot*

Who teaches you to shampoo? Is it not just a case of putting some shampoo on your head, lathering it, and washing it off?

Not necessarily. Try this Nutrigro® plan to stimulate hair growth through shampooing. Hair is fairly strong and can bear normal grooming. There is a correct technique for washing hair that has been used in India for centuries-follow it to keep your hair for longer.

How to shampoo:

1. **Brush hair before washing**
2. **Use a natural non harsh chemical shampoo**
3. **Wet the hair with warm water**
4. **Rub a small amount of shampoo in with your hands and cover your head with shampoo 2-3 times, start from the front working to nape of head with your finger tips**
5. **Wash off foam with warm water**
6. **Wash off hair with cold water**

7. **Massage your scalp-Ayurvedic Head Massage for 3-5 minutes**
8. **Dry your hair-blotting with a towel**
9. **Comb or brush hair after it has dried**
10. **Hair style-do not overstretch it**
11. **Use the right brush or comb- comb or brush it at least twice daily**

1. **Brushing hair before washing** can make loose flakes of sebum and dead skin build-up. Cleaning the scalp during shampooing would therefore be easier.

2. **Use a natural gentle shampoo. Even in shampoos that advertise as "natural", there are present quite often-harsh detergents.** These can strip away too much oil from the hair, causing shampoo residue to be left behind. Ingredients that help include Aloe Vera, Tea Tree Oil, Sage, Saw Palmetto, Nettle and non-Sodium Lauryl Sulphate detergent.

Choose a shampoo with a balanced pH; a level of 5.5 is ideal. The pH scale runs from 0 to 6.9 for acids and 7.1 to 14 for alkaline, with 7 being neutral. Generally conditioners are not as notorious as shampoos with respect to containing harsh chemicals.

Shampoos with conditioners included should be avoided. Shampoos and Conditioners serve two different functions. Combining the two diminishes the effectiveness of both.

• **3. Wet the hair with warm water to open up the pores and increase blood circulation in the scalp.**

- **4. Start shampooing from the front and going to the nape with your fingertips. Do not excessively shampoo** the hair as this can strip vital minerals like calcium, phosphorus, nitrogen and iron from the hair. When shampooing the hair, pour the shampoo into the hands **and rub the shampoo in with your hands rather than pouring it on your head**. Pouring shampoo directly into the hair may promote build-up in one particular patch.

- **5. Shampoo with warm water-** removing dirt and grease.

- **6. Rinse hair with cold water to open the pores and improve blood circulation.** Rinsing with cool water will help shrink the pores back to their normal size. After washing your hair or the thinning area with cold water run your scalp with your fingers deeply. Do this until you feel a tingling sensation in your scalp from the heat you are generating. The heat and rubbing activates the sebaceous glands. These energize blood flow-hence increasing the growth of new healthy hair-this is an old tried and tested method.

- **7. Massage the scalp gently with your fingertips to loosen flakes and build-up and to stimulate circulation.** Avoid using the fingernails as this may scratch the scalp and cause scarring over time.

In the 1940's Dr Lars Engstrand, a Swedish scientist, suggested that **pressure causes poor circulation to the arteries and to the smaller capillaries. This is why massage would help. He suggested that it is the thickening of the part of the scalp called the galea (top of head where head starts balding) that causes baldness in a number of people.** The galea is the part of the crown where male pattern baldness is seen.

It is for this reason that older balding men often have scalp skin that is more taut and more inelastic compared to a young person's. In early teens the galea is typically 0.2 millimetres but from the age of 16 to 55 the **size of the galea gradually becomes thicker. It also loses its elasticity.**

The result of this is that there is greater pressure and tension in this area. Hair follicles as a result do not receive the required nutrition for optimal hair growth. In time hair would eventually fall out. He also noticed that baldness is not seen further than half inch outside the galea. This is why men lose hair on the top of their scalp where the galea is and not from the sides and back. **Massage would help circulation.**

Massage comes from the Greek word massein, meaning, "to press gently". It is a way of removing toxins, soothing the body, relaxing and stimulating blood flow. Would it then not make sense to massage the scalp to increase blood circulation?

 Is there a technique to this or should one just use random manoeuvres?

No there is a specific secret ancient Himalayan Ayurvedic massage technique - see next Chapter on how to do the Ayurvedic Head massage.

- **8. After washing hair, dry the hair by blotting with a towel. Avoid rubbing, particularly with cloth towels.** This will pull hair when it is already in a weakened state due to the wetness.
- **9. Do not brush the hair when it is wet. Only after drying the hair, brush it.** Wetting hair helps straighten and detangle hair much better. However the stress on the hair shaft is increased.

- **10. Avoid overuse of hairstyles that pull the hair too tight** e.g. ponytails and braids. **These may cause traction alopecia or hair loss** especially along the sides of the scalp. Leave the hair chemically untreated for a time and leave it in a loose style may be a suitable remedy.
- **11. Your comb should be even and smooth toothed.** Your brush should have stiff and long bristles to increase blood circulation in the scalp.

Brushing the hair in general can be stimulating to the scalp. This helps encourage blood flow to the hair follicles. This helps in maintaining their health. A soft brush should only be used to make the hair shiny. **Comb your hair at least twice a day.** Do not over comb or over brush, as this will damage the hair. **Wash your hair not less than twice a week,** depending on how greasy or dirty it gets.

Which are the best dyes for people to use?

Semi-permanent hair colour or henna are better alternatives as these minimize the harsh reactions between the relaxer or perm and the ammonia and peroxide amounts in permanent dyes.

- It is always best to allow the hair to rest untreated as much as possible, and avoid mixing chemical processes. Follow the directions on all perms and relaxers. **Excessive colouring, styling or heat treatments and chemical treatments can damage hair.** Sometimes this may cause a breakage in the hair even though directions are followed. Do not use metallic hair-curlers as they make hair brittle. Perms and relaxers have harsh chemicals in them that chemically alter hair, and long-term use of these chemicals can cause harm to hair shafts and follicles causing some hair loss.

If you shampoo as above, including using hot and cold water, and massage the head you will be stimulating your scalp straight away.

Chapter 8

Himalayan secrets to give you healthy hair through ancient Ayurvedic head massage

"A massage a-day will keep the Aspirin away"
©Ravi Bhanot

Can a massage help in keeping your hair for longer?

Ayurvedic massage techniques have been used for centuries to promote hair retention and hair regrowth- how can the ancient Ayurvedic head massage technique help you?

• **The objective of this massage technique is to work on marma (Sanskrit for hidden) points on the skin and to work on the cranium rather than superficially just over the scalp.** A marma point is a place where two or more tissues meet (for example a muscle and tendon). We are a body of energy and wherever there is a blockage of energy health problems ensue. **Marma points are connected via** *nadhis* **(channels) to energy depots called Chakras. There are seven energy centres or Chakras that balance these energies through working on the endocrine glands. Endocrine glands are responsible for releasing hormones in the body. Hormones regulate the workings of the body .If we are happy it is because "happy" hormones have been released. Massaging marma points influences chakras and in this way rebalance energies in the body.**

- By massaging the cranium the scalp is relaxed, temperature is increased locally and the blood flow is increased. **This technique should be done daily irrespective of whether you are having a shower or not.** The best way to make this part of your life is to do it at a specific time-morning, evening when watching TV, at night or when showering (if you do this everyday). Make this a habit to keep your hair for longer. As with any massage technique take care and massage gently at first.

Technique:

- Step 1. **Massage the third eye** in a clockwise circular motion with medium or *rajasic* pressure 10 times and **repeat this movement across the left side and then the right side of the forehead.**

- Step 2. Then **using the same movement upwards from the side of the temples to the crown**, using both hands and same amount of pressure. **Then work towards the back of the neck.** By doing this you are massaging the same route that blood takes to return to the heart.

- Step 3. **Massage the *Brahmi* marma point with clockwise circular movements.** This point is 8 finger widths (your own) from the line of your eyebrows, on your scalp. You know you have hit this point when you feel a slight ridge here. Massage here clockwise 10 times.

Step 1

Step 2

Step 3

Step 4

Step 5

Step 6

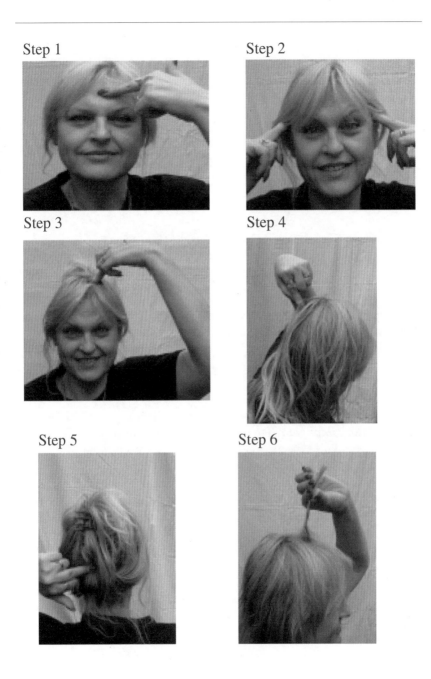

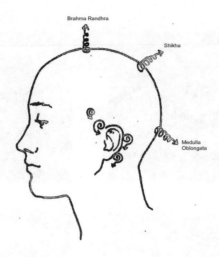

- Step 4. Then **massage with the same action 10 times at a marma point called the *Shikha*.** To locate it, bend the head forward so the chin touches the chest. This point is 8 finger widths from the medulla oblongata (the place where the skull meets the neck-see diagram below).

- Step 5. **Finally massage with the same technique 10 times at the *Medulla Oblongata*.** This point is at the centre back of the head where the skull meets the neck. It is responsible for the communication of the brain with the nervous system.

- Step 6. **Complete the massage by doing the following**:
Take a small amount of hair from the three-marma points, *Brahma Randhra*, *Shikha* and *Medulla Oblongata* and twist it. Gently pull each one starting from the *Brahma Randhra* and ending at the Medulla Oblongata.

 What if you cannot do this as you have little or no hair?
Do the steps you can!

If you just cannot manage this technique or cannot get this into your daily schedule then as second best you could lie on the edge of your bed with hanging your head over the side. This will help blood supply to the scalp of the head.

Alternatively learn the Ayurvedic Head Massage as a one-day workshop at The Ayurveda Institute of Europe. I co-founded this not-for-profit Institute so that Ayurvedic Massages would as common in Europe as they are in India. See www.ayurved-ainstitute.org for more details.

*We conducted a survey to see the effects of stimulating the Brahmi marma in people. We asked a group of people to shower their head including wetting the Brahmi marma and to a group of people not to wet this area. This area was covered with a thick towel or avoided. Virtually everyone who showered over this spot found they were far more invigorated after the shower than those who had not covered this area. Try it yourself and see if it works! **Please let me know your experience.***

Chapter 9

The *Nutrigro® Diet* Plan – How to energize your hair roots through food.

> *"Let food be your medicine and medicine be your food."* Hippocrates
>
> *Why would food have a bearing on hair loss especially those who would argue that it is really due to hereditary reasons? They may argue they eat exactly what their friends or family who have not got hair loss or hair thinning eat-so has food really got a bearing in hair thinning or hair loss?*

- We know that **hair cycles are genetically pre-programmed. We may only be able to influence the length of each cycle. We also know foods can affect Testosterone and Dihydrotestosterone (DHT) levels. Testosterone converts to DHT with the help of the enzyme 5-alpha-reductase. DHT shrinks hair follicles in men with the gene for male pattern baldness (MPB). Ultimately this results in the death of hair follicles and hair loss.** So if we **choose foods that influence this reaction in the body, we can influence how long we keep our hair for**. Most would agree that our body and hair would be healthier if our internal body was healthy too.

> *Nearly 30% of us die before we reach 65 and we have a less than 20% chance of living without cancer or heart disease. Why?*

Hair loss has increased drastically this century in both males and females. One main reason is our diet. **Snacking on 'fast foods' has increased greatly rather than eating wholesome balanced meals.**

- **The *Nutrigro®* Diet plan will help hair loss, hair thinning as well as overall health and vitality.** It is for those people who are healthy and who have no other health complaints.

- **The *Nutrigro®* Diet looks at four main food areas and what is ideal for us to eat: 1.sugar 2.salt 3.minerals 4.low fat and 5.appropriate diet for hair.**

- **1. Sugar Intake**

White sugar is refined and has all fibres, proteins and other nutrients stripped from it. After this it is bleached.

The body produces insulin to help the body's cells use glucose (sugar) for energy and to keep the blood sugar level down. **The amount of sugar taken influences how much insulin is released. If insulin levels are kept at a normal range, the body is able to control the production of the essential fatty acid, arachidonic acid** (1). **This acid has an influence on the production of Testosterone and hence on DHT** (2). **Arachidonic acid also controls the production of eicosanoids - hormones that control amongst other bodily systems, high blood pressure and production of keratin**, the component that makes 97% of hair. Keeping the diet balanced is the key-see later.

The amount of sugar consumed in the west has increased.

- **2. Salt**

It is medically accepted that an excess intake of **salt can increase blood pressure. Reduced blood vessels have an effect in their ability to deliver nutrients to the scalp.**

Preliminary studies have shown that eliminating salt from the diet helps reduce the rate of hair loss. An excess of salt has been linked to other hair conditions such as dry hair and dandruff. Our salt intake is thought to be ten to twenty times more than is required by the body.

There have been studies showing the correlation between salt intake, baldness and blood pressure. 20,000 men and women took part in a study carried out by Professor Peter Schnohr at University of Copenhagen in 1993. **He found that bald men had significantly higher heart attacks than men who still had their hair.**

The Physicians Health Study, involving 22,071 male Doctors over an eleven-year period, looked at the pattern of deaths and heart diseases and correlated this with hair baldness amongst the Doctors. The relative risk of heart disease or death was noted against different patterns of baldness. It was noted that there was a **35% greater chance of risk of heart disease or death in bald people compared to people with hair and** there was almost a **70% chance where the people were bald and already had high blood pressure.**

Further evidence of the ill effects of salt comes from comparing diets of different communities. Communities where salt intake is low for example in the Yanomano Indians of South America there is also a low incidence of high blood pressure. It is also true to say that these communities probably have a lower level of refined foods, less alcohol and stress and have more exercise and more fruits and vegetables in their diet.

> *Message: Do not add any extra salt to your meals. 6g (1 teaspoonful) a day –recommended daily amount.*

- **3. Minerals**

Firstly to follow a diet you need to understand how it works and what is happening in our body at a cellular level.

Cells need oxygen, water and nutrients. We get these nutrients from the food we eat.

Each cell needs to eat in its own right to work atoptimum performance. In other words each and every cell needs its own nutrition for best health.

Many of the foods we eat every day are not what our cells actually need. They make our cells sick. This in turn makes us sick.

Consider your inner environment of our body.

 If you were getting enough oxygen, water and nutrients to the red cells, would you be functioning more optimally and would your hair be getting more nutrition for growth?

Of course yes is the answer. But how...read on....

In our blood we have bacteria, yeast, fungi and mould. Most are not supposed to be there but our imbalanced internal environment supports them.

The pH of our blood and tissue is exactly 7.365- slightly alkaline. **The scale of pH is between 1 and 14 where 7 is neutral, below 7 is acidic and above 7 is alkaline. An even slightly acidic environment would cause different microorganisms to grow within us.** The further our internal environment is from pH 7.365 the more imbalanced we become.

 What has this got to do with hair loss or thinning you may be wondering?

Growing research over the last 20 years, by **microbiologists and biochemists such as** Dr. Robert Young and Dr.M.Mortimer**, indicates that an over acidic internal environment is the source of disease or unhealthiness**-be it in any part of the body including scalp. **Our acid/alkaline balance in the body is influenced by our diet, the chemicals we use, radiation and stress.** All these increase the internal acidic environment.

The secret then to keeping the hair we have and improve our scalp condition is to remain alkaline, internally. This is what The _Nutrigro®_ diet does.

The body works to balance the fragile internal acid-alkaline base. It has to as our blood can only function at a precise pH level. The scientists suggest that to **neutralise acid food, the blood begins to draw on its alkaline reserves (minerals)** from tissues, to compensate. Our body has a certain amount of alkaline minerals to meet emergencies. When there is not enough from our diet then the body takes them from wherever possible. Calcium is taken from the bone and Magnesium is taken from muscles (3). The consequence of this is that there are various symptoms that the body suffers from as a result. Eventually however the overbalance causes the extra acid to be stored. The immune system is relied upon to neutralise what it can. The rest is then sent back to the blood to be dealt with. The cycle restarts again as more minerals are required to balance this extra acid. This of course puts a strain on the liver, the kidneys and the lymphatic system.

Continued blood pH imbalance causes the body to dispose of the acids through the skin. The symptoms seen are eczema, acne, soreness, itchy scalp and inflamed skin sometimes of the scalp.

Dr Linus Pauling, the only person to win the Nobel Peace Prize twice, said in the 1950's **"you can trace every disease, every sickness and every ailment to a mineral deficiency"**. We hear a lot of our clients say:

 "But I eat well, how could I possibly be mineral or vitamin deficient?"

A nutrition imbalance test tells them otherwise.

The 1992 Earth Summit in Rio suggested that the world's soil had been significantly depleted of its minerals in the west. This implies that we are not getting anywhere near as much vitamins or minerals as we used to from the soil.

Scientists have concluded that high mineral levels in the body are necessary to reduce the widespread increase of cancer, heart disease, diabetes, arthritis, brittle, dull hair and hair loss (4). The reason is simple- in acidic conditions cells begin to mutate.

You may be wondering: where have these minerals gone? The growing plants use the minerals. Logically the soil should be replenished with the essential minerals that are required in the soil. Unfortunately that is not the case. **Only three essential minerals are put into the soil through fertilizers-Nitrogen, Potassium and Phosphate.**

Where is the proof that minerals are responsible for good health and indeed long healthy lives? Well see the typical hair of Asian people - Chinese, Japanese and Indian. Their diets are vegetable orientated and they benefit from soil that has not been over-farmed like that in the West. There could be the argument that there are *a number of other factors that should be taken into account.... but read on...*

In 1926 Sir Dr Robert McCarrison connected diet to health. The Hunza Community of Northern India/ Pakistan was studied because of their mineral rich environments and diet and extraordinarily long expectancy of life. Common diseases such as heart disease, diabetes and asthma were uncommon in this group. **The conclusion drawn was that mineral rich water and natural plant minerals were making the difference.** *(The cynics may well argue that they have less pollution and perhaps less stress there too. This may be true as well.)*

 Does eating organic food mean you will get the missing minerals?

Organic food may taste better but ultimately it is still coming from the same depleted soil, so the answer is no!

So it begs the question can we get all our minerals and vitamins from our diet?

A lot of scientists, including myself, believe probably not.

When I was a Community Pharmacist I was concerned how many people were on medication for chronic conditions. They religiously came in for their medication month in, month out. They were not being advised on life style changes or advice on better eating. We too had not been trained in this. **The NHS was not putting any real emphasis on preventative medicine. There was no financial help in obtaining nutritional advice, learning or practicing yoga or joining the gym or given any real funding for alternative medicine (herbal, aromatherapy, and reflexology) or creating the culture for healthier living.**

There was no improvement in health. On the contrary if anything. I used to think what are we doing with the health of Britain? Surely there has to be a better method of getting people to be healthier than these pill-pushing fire-fighting methods that are commonplace in the NHS. Of course this is necessary in many cases, but let's look at the whole picture! Whilst symptoms may have improved or better hidden, are people really getting healthier? What do you think?

Were there fewer cases of people suffering from thinning or losing hair? This clearly could not be hidden! The answer was no. Hippocrates once said: "Let your food be your medicine and medicine your food".

He was right - when we have a one-off headache for example is our body saying to us, " I am craving for an Aspirin?" or might it be a cry for water, or fresh air or reducing stress or might it be a signal that the body is in (dis) ease?

In 1996 I decided that we had to do more to make people healthier than what we were offering on the NHS. Boots the Chemist made us an offer and we took this to meaning it was time to take a stand for what we believed in. My wife Sushma and I left Community Pharmacy to venture into "natural" Pharmacy.

I did post-graduate studies in nutrition, stress management, homoeopathy, massage and training in Ayurveda. My wife, Sushma, did similar training.

We started the HASS Alternative Health Clinic and co-founded the Ayurvedic Institute of Europe. This is now probably the largest Institute in Britain teaching Therapists Ayurvedic Massages, Ayurvedic Nutrition and Stress Management. The Institute is a not-for-profit organization that teaches, carries out research into plant medication and alternative treatments. Our research has focused on hair, allergies, breathing and skin complaints in particular.

 Do you think we are using plants for medicinal purposes anywhere near enough their full potential?

No, we don't think so either.

- **Marine plants,** amongst others I have found, were an ideal **vegetable based vitamin, mineral and amino acid source.** They come from the rich lakes of South India. They along with other herbs such as Amla (Indian gooseberry), Fenugreek and Saw Palmetto were providing the nutrients required for hair growth. We were beginning to see positive results with our clients suffering from hair loss. A pH litmus urine or saliva test was also showing that the clients were becoming more alkaline with the *Nutrigro®* diet and supplementation.

How to test if your body is alkaline

The best time to test your pH is about one hour before a meal and two hours after a meal.

Saliva pH Test: The Dr.M.Morter pH test (5) is purely an indication rather than a scientific test.

Wet litmus Paper with your saliva. Although generally more acidic than blood, salivary pH mirrors the blood. It tells us what the body is retaining. It gives an idea of the health of the extracellular fluids (area outside cells) and the alkaline mineral reserves of the body. The optimal pH for saliva is 6.4 to 6.8. A reading lower than this is indicative of insufficient alkaline reserves. After eating a meal, the saliva pH should rise to 7.5 or more. You want your saliva staying between 6.5 and 7.5 all day for your body to be functioning within a healthy range.

Acidosis, a condition when there is an extended time in the acid pH state (less than 6.4), can result in conditions such as rheumatoid arthritis, diabetes, lupus, high blood pressure and hair loss. **(Email me at ravi@coolherbals.com for a free litmus paper.)**

Message to take away: Let 70% of your diet be alkaline vegetables

- **4. Low fat**

A diet high in fat, especially fat from animal products, is thought to reduce the amount of sex hormone binding globulin (SHBG)(6). This is a protein that binds to the male hormone, Testosterone, circulating in the bloodstream.

As a result there is more Testosterone available to be converted into DHT. Studies show that a low-fat or vegetarian diet has less Testosterone floating in the bloodstream.

A recent study showed very high concentrated fat levels in a large percentage of young people. Obesity is running at around 1 in 4 to 1 in 5 in young people. Signs are that premature hair loss; hair thinning and poor health are also on a spiral upwards.

Can you help the world change this?

Please share your knowledge about the Nutrigro® Plan with who ever can benefit- anyone who has some aliment, health condition or disease- at least the part of the Plan that is relevant!

In 1985 a Japanese Research showed that there was an increase in balding in Japanese men who had increased their westernised diet of more red meat. The Researcher Masumi Inaba suggested that an increase in saturated animal fat caused oil glands in the hair follicle to increase in size causing more DHT to be produced and hence more balding.

- **5. Appropriate diet for hair**

Any diet that is a challenge is unlikely to be kept on a long-term basis. **A diet needs to be staple foods that emphasise on foods that keep the blood-sugar level balanced, is low in fat, salt and sugar, and is rich in minerals. It also needs to have vitamins, protein, fibre, carbohydrates and omega-3 oils for healthy hair and for regrowth of hair.**

The secret to the diet is keeping a 70% alkaline diet emphasising on Pitta pacifying food.

 What does this mean?

This means simply keep your diet richer in fruits and particularly green vegetable salads and eat particular vegetables and fruits. From the food table in Appendix 1 (at back of book) *eat approximately 40-50% complex carbohydrates (salad), 25-30% protein and 25-30% monosaturated fats.*

So what are alkaline foods and what are acidic?

Alkaline foods (fruits and vegetables) are rich in minerals. They are essential for hair growth.

According to Dr. M. Morter in his research An Apple a Day? (1996) acids can be from cells or they can be natural. Acid made by cells as they die is physiological acid. This is a lot weaker than the acid produced from high acid producing foods. The physiological acid does not need to be neutralised with minerals before it is eliminated. It is lost from the body through breathing and through talking.

Acids from fruits are also easily removed, just in the same way as physiological acid. **Acids from acidic food however differ. These foods are generally high protein foods such as meat, fish and grains.**

 These foods need to be neutralised with minerals before they can be removed from the body through the kidneys or bowel. Why?

This is because blood needs to keep its tight pH of 7.34, so any acid foods need to be neutralised with alkaline minerals.

High protein foods leave an ash or residue, once neutralised in the body, which is acidic-Sulphur, Phosphoric acid and Chlorine. Fruits and vegetables leave an ash that is alkaline. The alkaline residue is mineral rich – Sodium and Potassium.

In summary, fruits are acidic by nature but form rich alkaline reserves and their wastes are easily removed from the body. It should be noted that there are always exceptions in both groups.

All foods have different values of acid and alkaline ash.

According to Ayurveda –the ancient Indian science- hair thinning and hair loss is due to an imbalance of energies in the body.

To fully understand The Nutrigro® Nutrition Plan you may want to understand the background behind Ayurvedic nutrition. It is not that important to understand the theory- more how to use it.

Theory of how the *Nutrigro*® Nutrition Plan works

- **In Ayurveda a person is seen as a unique individual made up of all the five primary elements.** The five elements are: **ether (space), air, fire, water, and earth.** If one looks at nature we find that this too is made up of these five elements. 70% earth is water, 30% land (earth), surrounded by air and space (area left when air is removed from a vacuum) and fire (from the sun). This is why we are considered part of the cosmic nature of life.

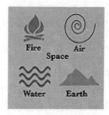

The food we eat and the weather around us are two examples of these elements. **Though we are made up of these five elements certain elements have an ability to mix together to create various physiological functions. Ether and air combine to form an energy that is known in Ayurveda as the Vata dosha**

Vata is responsible for the principle of movement. It can be seen as the force, which directs nerve impulses, blood circulation, respiration (breathing), and elimination (of waste). **When fire and water elements combine they form the Pitta dosha or energy. This dosha is responsible for the process of transformation or metabolism- breaking down of food into nutrients for example.**

Pitta energy is also responsible for metabolism in the organs, tissue systems and cellular metabolism, premature hair loss and hair thinning. When the elements water and earth combine they form the kapha dosha.

Kapha energy is responsible for growth and protection- stomach mucosal lining and cerebral-spinal fluid that protects the brain and spinal column are a type of Kapha energy.

Although each of us have all the three doshas or energies- the ratios of the doshas vary in each individual. This makes us all unique.

A **vata** person has more air and ether in them. This makes them usually thin and low in weight. He or she has thin, dry and rough skin. Vatas usually have curly, coarse and dry hair. Their appetites are variable and unpredictable. Vatas are hyperactive and can exhaust easily with restless minds that fantasise. They are light sleepers.

A **pitta** person has more water and fire. They have a medium height, build, and bone structure, with soft and oily skin. Pitta have hair that is soft and oily and will have a tendency to bald and grey early. Pittas sleep is short and deep.

A **kapha** person has more water and earth. They are usually large, big boned and strong. Kaphas have a tendency to be overweight. Kaphas hair is thick, wavy and greasy. Kaphas sleep deep and long.

The above is only a general guideline of a typical person's constitution. We are born as one Constitution-our natural - (*Prakuti*) and with time our constitution changes (*Vakriti*) due to factors such as age, environment and our food.

To enjoy the best of health, the aim is to get back to your original constitution (Prakuti). We all have these three energies although there may be more of one than another. The higher one is our primary dosha and the second highest one is our secondary. The permutations of the combinations are ten in total. One can have more vata than pitta energy for example-the primary dosha would then be vata and the secondary pitta. To work out your Body Constitution see an Ayurvedic Practitioner. (The Ayurvedic Practitioners Association website www.apa.uk.com) or fill in the questionnaire below or visit we-bsite www.ayurvedainstitute.org.

Answer the questions with someone who has known you for a long time to work out your life constitution. Answer, thinking how you have been throughout your life. Our life constitution has been determined at conception and this cannot change. Our present health balance (or imbalance) can be determined by answering how your health is at present. This can be changed.

*This questionnaire is not a diagnosis but gives you **some idea** about your Ayurvedic constitution. Tick one of the following answers. Then add up your answers. (How many 1, 2 or 3's did you get?)*

What is your Body Structure?
1 -Short, Thin, Weak
2 -Medium, Fleshy, Plump, Delicate
3 -Well proportioned, perfect, well-built

What is your Body Frame?
1 -Lean, Short
2 -Medium, Plump
3 -Large, well-built

What is your hair type: Body hair, beard or moustache?
1 -Scanty, Dry
2 -Scanty, Soft, tendency to grey hair or baldness or thinning
3 -Plentiful, Wavy, Glossy, Does not fall or grey prematurely

What is your skin like?
1 -Dry, Cracking, Rough
2 -Oily, Pimples, Freckles, Marks or blackheads
3 -Glossy, Clear, Smooth, Glorious, Fair

What are your nails like?
1 -Small, Blackish, Cracking, Breaking

2 -Small, Reddish, Smooth, Flat

3 -Big, Pinkish, Smooth, Glossy, Convex

What are your lips like?

1 -Blackish, Cracking, Shapeless

2 -Reddish, Smooth, Thick, Soft

3 -Pinkish, Smooth, Glossy, Proportionate

What are your teeth like?

1 -Very Small or Very Big, Cracking, Broken, Irregular

2 -Medium Size with gaps

3 -Even, Glazing, Straight, Smooth, Shiny White

What are your eyes like?

1 -White Part - Blackish or dark colour

2 -White Part: Reddish

3 -White Part - White

What is your normal body temperature?

1 -Less than Normal, Palms and Feet are cold

2 -More than Normal, Palms, Feet, Face and Forehead are Hot

3 -Normal, Palms and Feet are slightly cold

What are your joints like?

1 -Protuberant, Cracking, Unsteady

2 -Loose, Moderately Hidden

3 -Strong, Well Knit, Firm, Compact, Well Hidden

What are your Movements like?

1 -Unsteady

2 -Slow, Steady

What is your voice like?

1 -Rough, Hoarse, Weak, Dry

2 -Clear, Loud

3 -Deep, Pleasant, Soft, Charming

How do you talk?
1 -Very talkative, fast
2 -Talkative, impressive speaker, good at arguments
3 -Slow, Soft, Steady, Firm but talks little.

How much do you sweat?
1 -Normal
2 -Very easily and a lot, the body emits the foul smell of sweat

What is your appetite/ thirst like?
1 -Unpredictable, likes to eat fast.
2 -Good, has to eat after three to four hours, cannot tolerate hunger/thirst
3 -Comparatively less, can tolerate hunger/ thirst easily

What is the quantity of food and drinks that you consume?
1 -Not fixed, can vary
2 -Comparatively more
3 -Comparatively less

What sort of food do you prefer?
1 -Hot and Wet
2 -Cold or warm
3 -Hot and Dry

What are your stools like?
1 -Blackish, hard, once in a day
2 -Yellowish, Loose, once/twice a day

3 -Yellowish, well formed, once in a day

What is your sleep like?
1 -Less than six hours interrupted
2 -Six to eight hours, sound
3 -Eight hours or more, sound

What is your work strength?
1 -Get tired after small amount of work
2 -Moderate
3 -Good after doing large amount of work does not feel tired

How do you work?
1 -Fast, in a hurry
2 -Medium fast
3 -Steady, slow

What are your sexual desire and strength?
1 -Low
2 -Medium
3 -Abundant

What is your grasping (understanding) power?
1 -Sometimes grasps quickly, sometimes grasps late.
2 -Always grasps quickly and neatly, very clever, genius
3 -Always grasps late but understands best.

What is your nature?
1 -Jealous, timid, starts any work hastily sometimes aimlessly
2 -Short tempered, forgiving, self respecting, fearless, brave, very clever, good at decision making
3 -Grateful, brave, patient, not greedy, strong, calm, quiet, soft, withstanding physical and mental exertion, sharp memory, stable, thoughtful, generous, starts any work steadily and slowly

• **When any of the doshas (vata, pitta or kapha) accumulate in excess of our "norm" we need to reduce the dosha that has become excessive.** Herbal supplements may accelerate the process of removing these toxins. **Excess pitta energy in the sebaceous gland, at the root of the hair, or folliculitis can make the person start losing hair** (7). **We need to reduce or pacify the pitta energy.**

How many different tastes of foods are there and should we have them all in our diet?

The answer is yes whilst attempting to reduce the pitta energy.

Sweet - wheat, milk, dates, rice.
Sour - yoghurt, tamarind, lemon.
Salty - salt, kelp.
Pungent - onion, radish, chilly.
Bitter - bitter melon, rhubarb root.
Astringent - pomegranate, apples

- **In Ayurveda, hair is considered to be a by-product of bone formation. The tissues responsible for building bones are also responsible for the growth of hair.**

Which foods should be avoided as they increase pitta energy in the body?

Excessive intake of tea, coffee, salt, alcohol, meats (particularly red), pickles, yoghurt, cheese and excessive smoking. Eating too many fried, oily, greasy, spicy, sour and acidic foods also aggravates pitta.

To counteract pitta energy your diet should contain more green leafy vegetables, salads, milk, fruits and sprouts.

*Take more proteins, milk, buttermilk, cereals, yeast, wheat germ, soybean and vitamin A.

*Take cool or warm but not steaming hot foods

*Bitter, sweet, and astringent tastes

*Use less butter and added fat. Consume food with moderately heavy textures.

- Ensure that you maintain a regular bowel movement everyday. In case of constipation, a mild natural laxative can be taken. Triphala, an Ayurvedic herbal supplement, is useful.

- **Although we may have different doshas making our respective individual original constitutions the *Nutrigro®* diet would help rebalance energies.**

Message to take away: Eat 70% alkaline foods (fruits and vegetables), balanced with the six tastes of foods, emphasising on pitta reducing foods.

- The list in Appendix 1 (back of book) gives an indication of foods, which would be more beneficial. **The foods in the Pitta 'Yes' column are more suitable to eat than the ones that come up in the 'No' section unless they are modified in some way.** For example, having a little of something in the 'No' section with something a lot more of in the 'Yes' section. Note that Pitta dosha is characterized by fire or heat- so eating cooling foods would be more beneficial. It should be noted that this diet assumes that the person is healthy with no other health complaint.

- **Other health complaints may suggest aggravation of other energies in the body and it is a question of assessing which condition needs more attention in the first instance.** If there is a health complaint, visit an Ayurvedic Practitioner (visit The Ayurvedic Practitioners Association website www.apa.uk.com) or email me at ravi@coolherbals.com.

What does a diet for people having thin hair or losing hair need to have in it?

The 6 ingredients are Vitamins and Minerals, Protein, Fibre, Carbohydrates and Omega 3 oils

Role of Vitamins in hair loss

• **The word Vitamins** comes from the Latin word *vita* - meaning life. **Vitamins are needed for health, growth and maintaining body tissues. They are also required for the metabolism of other nutrients.** Most vitamins have to be obtained through food. Green vegetables are particularly alkaline and are a great source of vitamins and minerals. Raw vegetables have the advantage over cooked vegetables in that one does not lose some essential vitamins through cooking. **To pacify the *Pitta* dosha or energy, raw vegetables are more suitable than cooked, as they are more cooling** in nature-see Appendix 1 at back of book.

• **Protein is made up of amino acids.** Amino acids are naturally occurring nitrogenous organic acids that are found in plant and animal tissues. There are 22 amino acids that go to make thousands of proteins. Each protein performs a different function. Proteins can be divided into complete and incomplete proteins. Eating correctly is therefore important. **Proteins are needed for healthy hair and skin, as they are the building blocks for body tissue.** Protein is amazing as it is broken down to amino acids when digested and they become a protein again when they reach the body's cells. Proteins help in keeping the acid alkaline balance. Vegetables, fish and meat are sources of protein. Lentils, beans, soybeans are also good sources of protein.

- **Fibre adds bulk to food.** Fibre is available from vegetables, fruit, grains and whole grain bread.

- **Carbohydrates breakdown in the body to release energy.** They contain carbon, hydrogen and oxygen. If the energy is not needed it is stored in the liver as glycogen for later use. The liver can however only handle a certain amount. The rest is converted into fat. When the body needs more energy, the fat is converted back into glucose. High carbohydrate high fibre foods such as those seen in whole grains, vegetables, fruits and pastas are healthier than carbohydrates in the form of sweets, potato chips or sugared cereals.

Nutrient particles are carried to our cells via an electrical charge. Lifeless foods like processed foods, which are of low frequency, do not give the body the electrical energy it requires. The body needs to use up electrical nerve energy to make the digestive system digest these foods. Charges are measured in Mega Hertz (MHz) and typically range from 0 to 250+. Fruits carry energy of 63-73MHz and Green vegetables carry 70-90MHz. This is the sort of energy levels our head prefer. Eat more energetic live green fruits and vegetables!

- **Omega-3 fatty acids are polyunsaturated fatty acids** classified as essential because they cannot be synthesized in the body. They must be obtained from food. These increase oxidation and the digestion rate. They help transport minerals throughout the body. The "good" fats are Omega 3,6 and 9. Omega 6 too is vital for healthy hair for the above reasons. They are present in oils such as flax seed, olive oil, nuts such as almonds, pumpkin and sunflower seeds or branded oils such as *Udo's* oil.

- **Free Radicals- these are unstable oxygen molecules**. They lack one or more electrons and are therefore in search of other molecules in order to "steal" an electron from them and hence become stable. Research shows that free radicals accelerate the aging process. Our body produces some antioxidants but we need to take sufficient amounts regularly of antioxidant vitamins and minerals to counteract the work of free radicals.

Free radicals work on the scalp and hair to increase the cellular breakdown, ageing and high blood pressure.

Vitamins

- **Vitamin B5 is Pantothenic acid and B3 is Niacin. These are vital for hair growth.** Pantothenic acid is necessary for the well being of every body cell and neither carbohydrate nor fat can be changed into energy without it.

- **Biotin is a member of the vitamin B family. It plays a key role in the metabolism of proteins, fats and carbohydrates.**

- Biotin plays a key role in the growth and maintenance of hair, nails and bone. **Hair loss and brittle nails have been correlated with biotin deficiency** and these symptoms are often alleviated when optimal biotin levels are achieved. Biotin is found in milk, liver, whole grains, yeast and Vitamin B12 is available in unpolished rice, nuts, eggs and liver. **Choline is a vitamin B like nutrient that helps counteract the effects of stress.** Choline supplements prescribed to balding patients produced significant results.

- **Folic acid is a B Vitamin and helps blood formation and resistance to infections.**

Deficiency of folic acid can cause anaemia, which can lead to hair loss problems, weakness, tiredness, breathlessness, irritability or insomnia

Alcohol, contraceptive pills and some drugs reduce folic acid levels in the body.

- **Vitamin B12 is needed for cell production-particularly for red blood cells.**

How do you know you are deficient in Vitamin B12?
Look out for a smooth sore tongue, poor memory, tiredness, menstrual disorders (in women) or poor appetite. A deficiency could be due to pregnancy, vegetarianism, alcohol, smoking or parasites.

- Taking enough antioxidants such as Vitamin E, C, Beta Carotene and high fibre is essential. Vitamin E works better when taken with Vitamin C.

- Vitamin E is meant for stimulating the oxygen intake in the body and improving blood circulation. If there is good blood circulation, hair growth is enhanced. Vitamin E is found in vegetable oils and dried nuts.

Vitamin C assists the normal functioning of capillaries that carry the blood to the scalp. Vitamin C also helps in neutralising toxins and impurities in the body. It helps the absorption of iron from food. **This is essential to help food reach hair follicles and consequently for more natural hair growth.**

How do you know you are deficient in Vitamin C? Look out for dry rough skin, dry cracked lips, inflamed bleeding gums dry scalp, brittle hair, hair loss or weakness.

Certain drugs decrease our Vitamin C reserves or absorption-antibiotics, corticosteroids, anti-arthritis medications and oral contraceptive drugs. Alcohol, smoking, stress, gastric or duodenal ulcers and diabetes mellitus do not help either.

- **Vitamin E helps peripheral blood circulation.** It is found in tissue membranes in every cell of the body. Farmers give Vitamin E to their animals so that their animals may have thicker healthier fur.

Vitamin A also helps keep our hair healthy. It is present in cabbage, broccoli and spinach.

Minerals

- There are some minerals that are particularly important for hair growth and maintenance.

- **Iron.** This is a major mineral. It is required for making haemoglobin (a protein found in red blood corpuscles that carry around oxygen), certain enzymes and is **essential for the growth and maintenance of hair.** Oregon Health Sciences University found that seventy two percent of women in the premenopausal group were found to have iron deficiency as the cause of Telogen effluvium. (Telogen effluvium is an abnormal loss of hair usually due to a change in the normal hair cycle. Most of the hairs are normally in the growth stage but when Telogen effluvium occurs, a greater proportion of the hairs enter the resting phase of the cycle and hair shedding is greater than normal).

Iron deficiency is the most common cause of Telogen effluvium in premenopausal women whereas medication is the most common cause of Telogen effluvium in women who are postmenopausal.

Iron deficiency could also be the most likely underlying cause when hair loss is subtle over years. A deficiency in this mineral could be due to menstruation and pregnancy in women. Dr Michael Sharon, author of *Nutrients A-Z*, suggests that in one period, a woman will lose around 10-15 mg of iron and throughout a pregnancy around 600-1000mg will be lost.

In certain people lack of iron, in the diet, can lead to hypothyroidism. This in turn leads to an imbalance in minerals such as zinc and cooper. As a consequence the body starts to absorb toxic metals such as lead in larger amounts. Iron's absorption in the body is also reduced by foods that bind to iron-such as high fibre foods, spinach and chocolate and by drugs such as tetracycline, levodopa and methyldopa.

How do you know whether you are anaemic? Typical symptoms are:

- fatigue and weakness
- pale skin
- irritability
- decreased appetite
- feeling dizzy or light headed

A Ferritin blood test could confirm whether you are iron deficient.

The reduction of iron stores passes through three stages: lowered iron stores, iron depletion and iron deficiency anaemia.

1) **Lowered iron stores**: This is where **iron stores are reduced but not exhausted**. There are no clinical effects detected.

2) **Iron depletion**: This shows up in laboratory tests. Haemoglobin **concentration may be below 'normal'** for that person's reference range. If the person increases their iron intake the haemoglobin levels would rise.

3) **Iron deficiency anaemia**: This is where **no iron is left** remaining in the bone marrow. Haemoglobin production reduces to below the acceptable range for the body to function properly.

It is interesting to note **that iron deficiency can occur even if the person is not clinically anaemic** and has normal haemoglobin levels. It is the Ferritin levels in the body that count rather than blood iron. Why? This is because Ferritin is a protein that stores iron in the body. The serum ferritin level, the amount of ferritin in your blood, is directly proportional to the amount of iron stored in the body. Whereas Ferritin level tends to be constant blood iron level can vary with diet. The normal range of Ferritin in the blood is between 37-168 mcg/dl and you need at least it to be 70 mcg/dl for good hair growth.

So why are some people anaemic?

There may be a number of reasons: read on...

They may not be eating enough iron rich foods such as green leafy vegetables, nuts, red meat or cereals or it may be that the amount of iron absorbed is not sufficient. Taking Vitamin C when supplementing your diet with iron can actually help absorb iron into the blood stream more completely. Good sources of iron include cream of wheat, dried fruit, soybeans, red meat, tofu and broccoli.

It is estimated that only about 10% of ingested iron is absorbed into the blood each day depending on the type of food in the diet.

A decreased absorption of iron can be caused by medications that reduce stomach acids, chronic diarrhoea and partial removal of the intestines or stomach (gastrectomy). Some foods, such as coffee, bran, soybeans, split peas and dried beans can actually decrease the absorption of iron into the blood stream.

> *Message: Avoid tea until at least an hour after eating as it contains tannin. This interferes with iron absorption.*

4) Heavy periods

Heavy periods (menorrhagia) is a common cause of moderate anaemia in pre-menopausal women who have no other symptoms. Symptoms of anaemia include tiredness, lethargy, feeling faint, becoming easily breathless. One may look pale. About 1 in 10 women will become anaemic at some stage due to heavy periods.

Long-term (chronic) bleeding is the most common cause of iron loss that leads to iron deficiency.

Hair follicles contain ferritin. When the circulating stores of ferritin decline, then support for more essential cells is derived from hair follicles. This can affect the ability of the hair to grow. There is a development of vellus (non pigmented fine hairs). Seeing fine hairs could be early indication of deficiency of iron.

- **Iodine**

Iodine is necessary for hair growth. Sheep farmers found that grass in iodine-depleted soil seriously affected the growth of wool in their sheep. Likewise, to avoid hair loss, you need iodine. **Lack of iodine can cause hypothyroidism. In hypothyroidism cell metabolism slows down and body and hair cells do not receive the energy they need to function properly.** How can you check whether you are lacking iodine and hence possibly have hypothyroidism?

Check your thyroid with a mercury thermometer (not a digital thermometer). Place it in your underarm on awakening. Check the temperature. The normal body temperature for good thyroid function is 97.8 to 98.2 degrees F (36.5 to 36.7 degrees C). Take your temperature for 5 days. Menstruating women should start their 5-day check on Day 3 of their cycle.

If the temperature is below 97.6°F (36.4°C) for the 5 days consult your doctor.

If you want a thyroid function test done make sure you ask for the free thyroxine (T4) levels to be tested as well as the thyroid stimulating hormone (TSH) levels to be tested. If the T4 level is at a lower end of the range and the TSH levels at a higher this is a sign that the thyroid is not functioning as well as it could even though the laboratory may give your result as "normal". **If you are losing hair and your body temperature is continuously lower than 97.6°F (36.4°C) consider taking Iodine in your diet.** Iodine is found in seafood, eggs, potatoes and seaweed and in *Nutrigro®* Hair Food capsules. **Cut down on foods that reduce the uptake of iodine by the thyroid. These include: cabbage, cauliflower, mustard, sweet corn, peanuts and almonds.**

Hyperthyroidism can cause hair loss too. This is where the thyroid is over performing causing symptoms such as nervousness, sweating, weight loss, enlarged neck and hair loss. One cannot test for hyperthyroidism in the same way as described above (i.e. for hypothyroidism). Try the following: reduce the activity of your thyroid by eating the above listed foods-the opposite of what you do for hypothyroidism.

- **Calcium**

This is also a **component of nails and hair**. Some scientists believe that there is **a hair growth-promoting hormone made by the thyroid, called calcitonin gene-related peptide (CGRP). This hormone regulates calcium. So taking calcium may help promote hair growth through the production of this hormone as well as being a component of hair.**

- **Silica**

This is a trace mineral. **Silica provides strength to hair and stops hair breakage.** Silica works by stimulating cell metabolism and cell formation. This slows the ageing process. Foods that are rich in silica are rice, oats, lettuce, parsnips, asparagus, onion, strawberry, cabbage, cucumber, leek, sunflower seeds, celery, rhubarb and cauliflower. A lot of these foods are part of Asian diets. Asians tend to have strong and healthy hair.

- **Cobalt**

This mineral has to be obtained from a food source. It is a part of Vitamin B12. It is **essential for building red blood cells.**

- **Copper**

This mineral is **required to convert iron into haemoglobulin.** It helps the amino acid tyrosine to work as a pigmenting factor for the skin and hair.

- **Zinc**

Zinc is present in all cells and tissues. Its responsibility is to **help direct enzymes to digest better so that more nutrients reach the hair.** It oversees the processes in the body and it is an important antioxidant. **Zinc is what is called immunomodulator-it balances out immune responses. So in alopecia areata where the immune system is imbalanced, zinc helps calm down to reduce or stop the attack on hair follicles.** Zinc helps the immune system perform better too.

Zinc is also required for the best balance of the hormones Progesterone, Oestrogen and Testosterone. Zinc will help where a hormonal imbalance is the cause of hair loss or hair thinning.

How do you know you have a zinc deficiency?

Look out for signs such as eczema, mental apathy, hair loss, susceptibility to infections, and loss of sense of smell or taste.

There is a good possibility of zinc deficiency if you eat a high processed food diet because it is additive rich.

It is possible to test yourself to see if you are suffering from a zinc deficiency.

Add 5ml of a solution called the Zincatest solution to a 60ml glass of water and gargle with a small amount of the diluted mixture around in your mouth for about 10 seconds, after eating food. Then either swallow the mixture or spit it out. Check what taste you have in your mouth.

If you taste nothing, you have a serious zinc deficiency.
If you have a slightly dry, furry or even sweet taste in your mouth, you are low in zinc.

If you have a definite taste in your mouth, which intensifies with time, you have a reasonable level of zinc in your body, but still not enough.

If you get a strong unpleasant taste in your mouth, which you notice immediately, your zinc levels are fine.

The normal zinc levels are 11-24micromol/dl, but the minimum level for hair is at least 14. So make sure your levels are not just in the normal range but are actually high enough for good hair growth. For a Zincatest visit www.lambertsvitamins.co.uk

- **Selenium**

This mineral is also an antioxidant. **It works synergistically with Vitamin E** (the two together are more effective than separately).

- **Magnesium**

Magnesium is essential for the functioning of the heart and liver, good nerve and muscle function, balanced metabolism and strong bones. **It helps in the production and repair of cells and is necessary for Calcium absorption and of Vitamin B1 and B6 metabolism. All these of course are required for healthy hair growth and to stop hair loss.**

The above vital food components can be obtained from the foods listed in Appendix 1.

This is only a guideline - you may need to see an Ayurvedic Practitioner for individual consultation if you have any health problems.

- **Mineral water has minerals in it and is a better source of water than tap water.**

 How much water should one drink daily?

As a male adult we need to be drinking –2-2.5 litres of water daily and as a woman 1.5 litres of water.

Why? If we are 70% water based we need to replenish water fluids lost through sweat and in the process of removing waste from the body.

It does not help drinking diuretics such as tea, coffee and alcohol as these cause more water to be lost from the body than are replenished.

Virtually every client we have seen in our Clinic suffering from a hair thinning, hair loss or a scalp problem has been dehydrated.

It is estimated that in Europe and America 70% plus people are dehydrated most of the time. This does not help the best growth of hair.

Why is water necessary for growth of hair?

This is because blood is predominantly made up of water and this brings nutrients to the scalp. Blood also takes away toxins and waste products from the scalp. Nerve impulses need water as a conductor to convey information and improve the activity of organs and it is also needed to detoxify the liver and kidneys and rebalance hormones.

How can you drink so much water a day?

Drink from a pint size (about half litre) glass and at scheduled times. - Maybe when you wake up, mid-day, mid-afternoon and last thing at night.

- **It is best to drink one hour before or after food.** If you are trying to slim, fill your stomach with water prior to eating. For everyone else avoid drinking just after eating. This is because water dilutes the enzymes (natural chemicals in our body that quicken processes in the body) required to digest food.

Eating a high content of water-rich foods is a way of increasing water intake. These should make 70% of your diet. Why? This amount allows the body to cleanse itself rather than being clogged up Lettuce is 96% water, broccoli or carrots 91%, oranges 88%, bananas 76%, cheese 40%, bread 36%, nuts 5%, dry cereal 4%, white sugar virtually 0% and oils 0%.

Message to take away: Do not be dehydrated. Keep up the water intake.

How can you check whether you are dehydrated?

Are your lips usually dry (allow for the weather)?

Check the colour of your early morning urine. Usually the darker shade of yellow is an indication of dehydration.

Drink one litre of water on an empty stomach and see the colour of urine that you pass. It will almost definitely be a very light yellow shade unless there is interference from foods or medicine you may have taken in the previous 24 hours.

When pinching the back of your hand how quickly does it take for the skin to come back to its normal self?

Are you prone to being constipated?

At the Clinic we use a *Bodystat* Body Mass-measuring device. We put an electrode on one side of the foot and one on the hand and we pass a light current through these electrodes. The greater the fat content and extent of dehydration, the longer it takes for the current to flow through. At home you can buy relatively less inexpensive Body Mass Index devices to measure your Body Mass Index and your level of dehydration.

- **Stop or cut down on smoking.** Smoking affects blood circulation. The habit kills approximately 1 in 6 people and is a preventable cause of death. Cigarettes contain Nicotine and Carbon Monoxide amongst other chemicals. Nicotine is a stimulator. It stimulates the stress hormone, adrenalin, to increase the heart rate and blood pressure. Carbon Monoxide affects the amount of oxygen blood can carry around to the heart. **The effect of stimulating the blood vessels and increasing the pressure on the heart's pumping action means a restriction in circulation.**

Nutrigro® Supplementation

There are various minerals and vitamins required for healthy hair.

It is not always possible to have every component required for excellent health and hair - either it is not taken in the diet or enough is not taken in. A supplement can therefore be helpful.

- The products I have formulated **contain marine-based nutrients - in the male formulation there is refined marine proteins, natural iron, vitamins and minerals required for healthy hair. I have also added a traditional herb known to help hair - Saw Palmetto.**

- Three formulations are made-one for males and two for females. This is because the requirements of males and female are different. **There are two female versions-one for most women with nutritional needs for healthy hair and one for women needing an oestrogen supplement.**

- As discussed earlier **Saw Palmetto is useful in slowing the process of Testosterone to DHT. By inhibiting this process hair loss can be prevented or at least kept to a minimum as mentioned earlier. This is particularly useful for men.**

In place of Saw Palmetto **in the women's formulation we have added the herb Amla.**

Amla or **Indian Gooseberry is a very rich source of Vitamin C. It has been traditionally used in India for centuries to keep healthy hair. It is of cold potency and helps in suppressing *Pitta* dosha (energy constitution). According to Indian medicine the imbalance of this energy is one of the main culprits in causing hair loss and premature greying of hairs.** Amla works on improving liver function and digestion. This helps growth of hair. Amla or Indian gooseberry (Phllanthus embilica) is a fruit that matures in the autumn. **Amla has been traditionally used in India for centuries for hair growth and pigmentation.** It is rich in the antioxidant Vitamin C. **Research suggests that it rejuvenates hairs and prevents split ends.**

• **Fenugreek (methi) has been used in India, Egypt and in Greece traditionally for long healthy hair.** Fenugreek is understood to **increase the blood vessel size to the scalp. The improved blood circulation improves nutrient supply to the scalp. Fenugreek is rich in vitamins, minerals, iron and calcium** in their natural organic forms. The body easily assimilates these.

Methi (fenugreek) is a commonly used ingredient in Indian recipes and is consumed in both its forms -leaf and seed. The leaves are bitter, but when tender the bitterness is subdued. The seeds are powdered or used as whole spices in marinating and in curries.

Fenugreek seeds are nourishing and rejuvenating. They are also stimulating. The seeds are a digestive aid in cases of abdominal distention, gas, malabsorption, pain and heaviness in the stomach. Fenugreek cleanses and detoxifies the body by drawing out waste matter and expelling it.

- **Refined marine plants** found in **natural alkaline lakes are about 70 percent** *complete* **protein, with all the essential amino acids in perfect balance.** They also have vitamin B12, carbohydrates, rhamnose and glycogen. These give the body quick energy without taxing the pancreas.

- **Around 7% fatty acids - almost all these are essential fatty acids, linoleic acid and alpha-linoleic acid are present too.** Essential fatty acids produce hormone-like substances that regulate functions such as blood pressure, the immune system and inflammation.

- **Natural Iron -a biochelated organic iron is present too. This is about 50 times richer than seen in raw spinach and 28 times richer than in raw beef liver.** This is better absorbed than the chemical iron present in the array of iron preparations available.

Hormonal imbalance

- **As women are approaching certain phases of life such as menopause, post-pregnancy or sometimes an unexplained hormonal imbalance, the natural production of hormones, estrogens and progesterone reduces. This leaves the scalp hair more prone to the effects of male hormones- the androgens. There is sometimes androgenetic hair loss and other undesired menopausal symptoms.**

A treatment for menopausal symptoms is HRT-Hormone replacement therapy- available on prescription. There have always been safety issues over the long-term side –effects of HRT. Research shows that synthetic estrogens can worsen hair loss in some cases. **This is partly because estrogen replacement increases the hormone prolactin. This in itself can cause hair loss or make hair loss worse.** It is not surprising to see that there is a trend turning to plant-based extracts as a natural alternative.

- A six-month Brazilian study assessed **the effects of plant based soy estrogen. 85% of the female subjects saw a significant improvement in menopausal symptoms including hair loss**, while 75% of them had lower cholesterol levels. The plant contains estrogen-like compounds called isoflavones.

 What has soy got in it?

There are four families of phytoestrogens (phyto means plant estrogens means female hormones) - isoflavanoids, stilbenes, lignans, and coumenstans. Don't worry if you don't remember these words-this is only for the passionate or scientists amongst you- it is more important to understand what these plant based chemicals do in our body.

Soy is one of the best-known sources of phytoestrogens as it has the isoflavones genistein, daidzein, and glycitein. Genistein and daidzein are among the most extensively studied of the phytoestrogens.

Do Asians who have adapted to a more western diet from their traditional high-soy diet have a greater issue of hair loss?

Yes - this was shown in research carried out in Japan (8)

Interestingly it has been shown by some researchers that women with higher levels of phytoestrogens in their diet are less likely to develop breast cancer.

Further supporting evidence that plants such as soy and green tea extracts help in hair loss came from research carried out by

Starka L and Co. (Czech Republic). **They showed that people with AGA (androgentic alopecia) have lower circulating levels of sex hormone binding globulin (SHBG) compared to the non-balding controls (9). Soy isoflavones elevate SHBG levels and help keep hair for longer.**

Ensure you have soy in your diet-this would help too. See the *Nutrigro® Diet* plan (Appendix 1 at the back of this book.)

Case Study

Jennifer an afro-Caribbean 32-year-old woman came to see me. Jennifer was losing hair profusely. Her medical history indicated that she had heavy periods, suffered severe PMT and that the pill did not suit her-particularly the oestrogen rich Marvelon or Dianette. She had also been told that she had a low SHBG- Sex Hormone Binding Globulin (a protein that binds to testosterone and so reduces the effect of testosterone on the scalp-quite often seen in women suffering from polycystic ovary syndrome, hypothyroidism and diabetes).

She was anxious that she might go bald. I was convinced that she would not - and that without taking drugs. I told her to take two capsules daily of the Nutrigro® Women's Hair Food Plus capsules along with using the Nutrigro® Serum, Shampoo and Conditioner. (The Hair Food Plus is a soy supplement. This helps when there is a hormonal imbalance in the body). Within six weeks she virtually stopped losing her hair. She is now on a maintenance dose of the capsules. Treat the cause not the symptom!

I know this was a long chapter but if you understand food you can make an enormous difference to your hair and scalp. Email me at ravi@coolherbals.com for a free pH test to see how alkaline you are.

Chapter 10- Nutrigro® Plan

See yourself with a headful of hair!

> *"If you want to know why you look today as you do, look at your past thoughts. If you want to know how you will look tomorrow, look at today's thoughts"* is an ancient Ayurvedic philosophy.

The mind controls the brain, if it is consciously applied and the brain controls the actions of the body. It follows that if we can control our mind our body would function better. It must therefore be fed the right thoughts.

This does not mean that if you go around saying "no weeds, no weeds" there wouldn't be in the garden- it means that we **have to consciously be positive that favourable results would ensue doing the** *Nutrigro®* **Hair Programme.**

How do you tackle the mind –try this:

1. **Let out your feelings – If you are stressed or feeling negative about your hair call a friend or join a group.** If you have not got a group, you can join locally by finding a community on the Internet. Contact me at ravi@coolherbals.com for advice or an indication of where help may be available. Otherwise there is always your Doctor or Counsellor.

2. **Visualisation and affirmation – Before going to sleep every night visualise the type of hair you would want to have. In bed close your eyes look about 30 degrees (2 o' clock position of a clock) in an upward direction.** It is thought that we look at the future in an optimistic light doing this. **Make the vision in colour- bright, large and alive-almost as though you**

could touch, feel and see it. Add as much clarity to it as you can- include the colour of the hair you would like, its texture, thickness and style. If you are struggling with this- just remember it is only a dream, a goal. Remember a belief is strong but a conviction has more certainty-that is what it must be!

 How are you going to reach a goal if you do not know what your goal is?

You aren't. A man once asked another man "where are you going?" "I don't know", the other man replied. "Well then it doesn't matter which road you take"

Don't think that your vision or dream is impossible or not unrealistic and therefore what is the point, trust the Universe!

 What does trust the universe mean?

If you say you are going to wake up at a certain hour in the morning-isn't it amazing that you can wake up at this time-unless you don't trust yourself and the Universe. In this case you would rely on an alarm clock or someone else and guess what, you will start losing confidence and trust in yourself and the Universe.

Dream of your vision last thing before sleeping. Affirm to yourself, ideally speaking aloud "I have lovely healthy, strong hair." Or your affirmation could be:

"I am grateful I have the hair I do" or it could be:

"My hair is growing stronger, thicker and healthier every day".

Some people find it helpful to have a photo or picture of how they would like to look like stuck somewhere they can see everyday, like on a cupboard door or on their computer. Do not worry about your goal. Allow your subconscious to help you reach your goal.

> *Remember how you communicate with yourself is more important than how you communicate with the world.*

3. Relax more – Find an activity that makes you feel happy. If you don't know what they are make a list of possible activities, even small ones such as reading. **Try laughing more as a way of relaxing.**

4. Associate with happy people or those who have a positive outlook to life. Read books and articles that are positive in nature. Going to self-development seminars can help too. For advice on which courses may help email me at ravi@coolherbals.com.

5. Write out your complaints or troubles on one page and on the other side of the page write the answer(s) to your problem. It is amazing how resourceful we are. If you can't think of the answers have some fresh air before writing, sleep on it or ask some friends for their opinions. Otherwise there is always professional help (1).

6. Have a Massage – I have shown earlier how to give an Ayurvedic Head Massage. If you do not want to give one to yourself perhaps a friend could help. Alternatively get a professional massage. **To find a masseur visit www.ayurvedainstitute.org, check in your local telephone directory or do an Internet search for a list**

of Therapists. Massage therapy can relax muscles and increase blood flow to skin and muscles. This would also help relieve mental and emotional stress. **Have a colonic irrigation every six months** to keep your bowels clear.

7. **Learn to say no** when you don't want to do something or you have imposed unrealistic demands on yourself. Be honest with yourself.

8. **It is not what you say but how you say it**-learn to say something effectively without offending others or feeling ignored.

9.**You can only change yourself** – avoid saying or thinking "if only he, if only she, if only they". **Rather think more "what can I change about myself to make my situation better."**

10. **Sometimes accepting** that things are the way they are and you cannot do anything about the situation helps.

> *Message to take away: Stress is part of life and it is how you handle it that counts. Use some of the above tips not only for healthier hair, but healthier life!*

Chapter 11

Nutrigro® Plan– Exercise to give you healthier hair

 "Exercise the body and you have exercised the hair and scalp"© -Ravi Bhanot

How can exercise help keep hair?

Exercising increases blood circulation, stamina and energy as well. It maintains strength in the bones and in the muscles. It will help clear the channels of the body so that all tissues can be thoroughly cleansed. An increase in blood flow to the hair follicles will help give nutrients to the head and scalp. Exercises help you eat better, digest better and eliminate waste better (1).

• Exercising promotes the production of hormones called endorphins. These make us feel "happier". **Exercises reduce stress and bring calmness to the body.** As mentioned before stress is also caused by the attack of free radicals in our body.

Stress releases adrenaline (the stress hormone) causing the heart rate to increase, the breathing to increase and blood pressure to rise. The liver increases the output of sugar and blood flow is diverted to the brain and large muscles. These free radicals are unstable molecules that increase oxidation in the body. In time this would cause an increase in the rate of ageing in the body.

- **When the body is excessively stressed the body loses large amounts of vitamins, minerals and protein (in the form of nitrogen) in the urine.** The sudden loss of nutrients is considered to be **one of the reasons for hair loss in stress related hair loss**.

So like so much in life, even exercise needs to be in balance.

Ideally how much exercise does one need to do?

20 minutes three times a week is recommended by a lot of professionals-but even some is better than none.

The first answer is not excessively. Too much exercise has been shown to increase the amount of a chemical called Pentane in the body. Pentane levels are known to increase when there is an increase of free radicals in the body. So how much is adequate exercising?

There are four types of exercises: **isometric, isotonic, naerobic and aerobic.**

- Isometric exercises-"iso" means same and "metric" means distance- is an exercise that has movement but no change in angle of joint. For example- pressing the palms together in front of one's body. This does **not demand much oxygen.**

- **Isotonic exercises-** is an exercise that has movement but has a change in angle of joint. Weight lifting is one such type of **exercise but again this may not improve blood supply to the scalp.**

- In **Anaerobic exercises the lungs and heart cannot meet the demand of the oxygen that is needed and refers to exercise that produces a short burst of energy.** This causes the person to stop to recover- after long distance running for example. **By exercising anaerobically, we burn glycogen as our primary source of fuel whilst the body stores fat.**

- In **Anaerobic exercises the lungs and heart cannot meet the demand of the oxygen that is needed and refers to exercise that produces a short burst of energy.** This causes the person to stop to recover- after long distance running for example. **By exercising anaerobically, we burn glycogen as our primary source of fuel whilst the body stores fat.**

- In **Aerobic exercises, demand for oxygen is not intolerable.** This results in the lungs becoming more efficient and the heart stronger. More oxygen is delivered to the scalp with nourishment to body cells. In combination with other food, the body produces energy. **15 to 20 minutes of vigorous exercises is required to get the optimum heart rate.** For less vigorous exercises such as walks, the exercises may have to be for longer.
Aerobic is a great way of exercising. If we condition our metabolism to work aerobically too by giving it the alkaline diet and aerobic exercises, our bodies would burn fat as the primary fuel.

- So **what is the maximum heart rate for an individual?** There is a simple formula **to work this out. 220 minus your age will give you your maximum heart rate.** So for a 30 year old this will be 190. **Your aerobic heart rate is this figure minus your age**- so 160 for this person. If you are recovering from a serious health condition, deduct 10 points and if you have a minor condition subtract 5 points.

To work out the minimum aerobic heart rate subtract 10 points from the aerobic heart rate. So for a 30-year-old person the maximum heart rate is 190. The maximum aerobic heart rate is 190-30= 160 and the minimum is 160-10 = 150. So the aerobic range is 150-160.

> *Does it matter which exercise you do?*
>
> *Not really as long as you are keeping within your aerobic range for 15-20 minutes.*

The best thing is you enjoy the activity - whether this is going to the gym, swimming or running. A particular favourite of mine is a rebounder (a mini trampoline). This strengthens, builds physical strength to cells, increases lymphatic drainage and increases the cells with oxygen. Cells are able to convert glucose into ATP and also glycogen. This glycogen can be stored for use for when a sudden need of energy is required.

> *Which exercises should you do for having healthier hair?*
>
> *The choice is yours.*

Another exercise that is vitally important to remove toxins from the body is this:

Vigorously brush all parts of your tongue first thing every morning after brushing your teeth until you feel you are about to bring something up. Just like parts of your feet have marma points relating to the major organs so does the tongue. Massaging the tongue will help remove toxins from all over the body.

Chapter 12

The Nutrigro® Plan: **How to use the art of breathing for healthier hair-using an ancient Sanskrit technique**

 "If we are programmed for only so many hair cycles or so many breaths shouldn't we be taking longer breaths? © Ravi Bhanot

• We breathe around 30,000 times a day and according to the World Health Organization (WHO) **normal breathing is 8 to 12 breaths per minute. At this rate the balance between oxygen and carbon dioxide are in balance and we feel in good health.**

Breathing through our nose keeps the amount of oxygen breathed in and carbon dioxide breathed out in balance. If we breathe through our mouths however as a normal way of breathing, we usually inhale and exhale air quickly in large volumes at a time. This can lead to a type of hyperventilation (breathing faster than we need to).

Research has shown that if we release carbon dioxide too quickly, the blood vessels that take blood to our cells constrict and the oxygen in our blood is unable to reach the cells in sufficient quantity (1).

• This includes the arteries, which carry blood and oxygen to the brain (the carotid). **Lack of oxygen in cells of the brain can switch on our sympathetic nervous system.** This brings our "fight or flight" response. We become tense, anxious, irritable, and possibly depressed.

- The body has to be in peak state. **All systems that are not necessary shut down in the body. All blood is directed away from the digestive or immune system as well as from the scalp and is directed to our arms and legs.** Over a regular and prolonged period of time this can be unhealthy for the hair. In a non-threatening fight or flight scenario this is called stress. In this state people are susceptible to hair loss and premature greying of hair.

- Consider also how oxygen and carbon dioxide are exchanged in the blood. Oxygen is carried in the blood via a protein called haemoglobulin. For oxygen to be released into tissues there has to be a certain amount of carbon dioxide.

If breathing is not balanced and there is too much carbon dioxide around in the blood the oxygen will not be released from the haemoglobulin. Tissues would suffer. Typical symptoms may well be tiredness and dark rings under the eyes.

- **Hair roots need oxygen and nourishment for healthy hair.** Keeping carbon dioxide levels normal is therefore important.

> *Take away message: Breathe through your nose.*

- **Why do we need oxygen for more hair?**
Human life depends on five main elements -
oxygen, water, nutrients, exercise and removing drugs from our life as much as possible. These are all needed in the right amounts. Without oxygen we could only survive for a few minutes.

- Oxygen is available in abundance. We can take in as much or as little as we want to keep us going. **It is estimated that we only use half the power that oxygen could give us. This is primarily because we do not breathe as efficiently as we could.**

- *How can we breathe more efficiently then?* **Firstly not by the autopilot method that we do-that is to say using only our autonomic nervous system.** We have a choice in consciously taking breathing in our own hands. Ignorance or laziness may be reasons why we are not adapting more efficient methods to breathing better.

- Our lungs have receptors, which take in oxygen. This is then distributed throughout the body. **Normal breathing fills up only half to two thirds of the lungs-primarily the top of the lungs. Most of the receptors are however at the bottom part of the lungs.** We are therefore not filling up with as much oxygen as we could. The air in the bottom part is therefore more stagnant and is richer with carbon dioxide. As explained above we can see the detrimental effect this is going to have on our hair. **Another interesting thought is it is estimated that that 90% of our energy comes from the oxygen we breathe rather than the food we eat and that around 70-80% of our waste by-products are eliminated through our breathing and our skin!** (2)

How to breathe better for healthier hair:
The *trigro*®Ancient Breathing System

When you **concentrate on regulating your breathing, the mind has less time to think negative thoughts and stress.** This as explained above, makes you hyperventilate and reduces the oxygen required received by the scalp.

Exercise 1

Try the 4-2-8 system of breathing. It is the type of breathing that you do when you are sleeping-a natural movement.

Nutrigro® **Ancient Breathing System**

* **Close one nostril with the finger, breathe in through the other.** Relax your ribcage and let your stomach out.

* **Fill your abdomen with air.** You could try this initially lying down to get it right. Place a book on your stomach. Breathe deeply, allowing your abdomen to expand. Watch the book move up and down. **Count till 4.**

* **Close both nostrils. Hold for 2.**

* **Open the previously closed nostril, close the other nostril and exhale slowly using your stomach muscles to force air out of the abdomen area and out through the nose. Count till 8.**

Now breathe in through the open nostril and repeat the above.

Repeat this 10 times at least once a day in the morning and ideally at night too. Your hair and scalp would appreciate it!

Exercise 2

Force air out through both nostrils with the stomach going in as you do so. Do this quickly at a rate of about one every 2 seconds. Repeat times 10, at least once a day in the morning and ideally at night too.

If all cells particularly the ones in the scalp require oxygen how else can we get more oxygen? The answer is drinking more water. In the Indian science called Ayurveda (*Ayur* means life and *Veda* means knowledge) it is thought that like the cosmos around us **we are made up of five elements-air, ether (space), earth, fire and water. Just like our planet we are made up of around 70% water.** It is almost like these cells, **around seventy trillion of them, afloat in a pool of water. If we do not drink enough water how would these cells survive** Oxygen is carried in haemoglobulin in the blood. **If the blood is sluggish due to lack of water, how is oxygen going to be carried around into the heart, liver, kidneys or skin?** Will you be doing any favours to your heart pumping system and to keeping blood pressure low if your blood is sluggish?

In our HASS Clinic I carry out a 'live blood' test to see the internal state of the blood. This test has changed the lives of thousands of people. A pinprick of blood is taken from the finger put on a slide and is examined under an electron microscope at 10,000 times magnification. The client sees the results on a monitor. You see the red blood cells either clumped up against each other, when one is dehydrated, or you see them floating separately as big round independent entities in a free flowing river, representing healthy blood and hence a healthy individual.

Research carried out by Dr. Batmanghelidji in Iran in 1979 (*Body's many cries for water?*) **showed that dehydration is a major reason for many illnesses including skin and hair.** He concluded that one should:

• Drink water regularly (never leaving a thirst unquenched)
• Every major organ in the body is desperate for water

Message: Drink water daily. If you are not reaching anywhere near the quantities recommended slowly, build up the volume on a daily basis. Drink from a pint size glass and schedule when you are going to drink your daily intake of water. Make a note in a diary, or mentally monitor the amount of water you are drinking. Breathe yourself to better health and hair – by the 4-2-8 system

Chapter 13

Find out your personal reason for hair loss- which hair-loss person are you?

In an Independent User trial, 15 volunteers used the *Nutrigro®* Hair system and took two of the *Nutrigro®* Hair supplements daily. In less than 8 weeks 65% felt that their hair appeared fuller and around 50% felt there was an improvement in the strength of their hair and that there was a reduction in the number of hairs that they were losing. A similar number felt that their hair was healthier. It should be stressed that this trial acted only as an indicator rather than being statistically complete. A number of tests have been carried out to test the effectiveness of the ingredients in the *Nutrigro®* products.

Below are live case studies that we have treated. Which one are you?

Post Pregnancy hormonal?

Case Study-Sharon

I am 36 years and I have suffered from thinning hair for about 9 months following the birth of my first baby. It was suspected that it could have been a postnatal hormonal problem, however mine was pretty bad. I had handfuls of hair falling out every time I washed or brushed my hair. This then stopped, leaving me with a dramatic hair loss compared to my previously very thick hair. This came at a particularly difficult time in terms of my body image. My hair was beautiful pre-pregnancy and during my pregnancy. The thinning took its toll on my confidence. It meant styling my hair to try and cover the problem took precious time I didn't have. Once the hair started growing back the problems continued. The new hair was very fine, along the hairline and looked like a nasty mistake at the hairdressers. Since using Nutrigro® Hair system it has much improved my scalp and made a difference to the hair looking full and healthier.

Hormonal Imbalance?

Case Study – Prem

I am 67 and I started to lose hair diffusely over my scalp. This was thought to be due to a hormonal or nutrition imbalance. I went to my Doctor and he prescribed a shampoo. This did not help. Taking the Nutrigro® Hair Food capsules, Nutrigro® hair Food Capsules Plus and Nutrigro® Hair System has made my hair stronger and I am not losing hair as I used to. Some new hair has started growing too.

Hereditary?

Case Study-Anne

I am a 58-year-old female with thin hair, possibly hereditary. My hair loss has got worse as the years have gone along. I have always been very aware of my poor hair and this has made me very withdrawn in company. My poor hair left me lacking in confidence outside my family unit. Despite keeping it well trimmed and clean I never felt it was my crowning glory. I even contemplated buying a wig on occasions but felt that I would be laughed at if I suddenly had a full head of hair.

I always kept my hair cropped short, visiting the hairdressers every 6 weeks for it to be trimmed but yearned to grow it a bit longer. After using Nutrigro® Hair System I began to grow out my hair. My hairdresser commented that my hair looked thicker at my last visit. My husband noticed small hairs, which appear to be new growth appearing.

I almost immediately noticed my hair loss was reduced using Nutrigro® products. My hair felt thicker, looked healthier and it seemed to start new growth. I had never invested in any "miracle cure" before, as I honestly believed that nothing would help, however, Nutrigro® has been a success as far as I can tell.

Diet?

Unknown reason?

Stress?

Case Study-Susanne

It was a stressful time of my life, my marriage broke up and my hair started to fall out. This was six years ago when I was 35. I had to stop using hair colour and too many heated styling aids. I found this difficult as I was at a time when I wanted to start going out and meeting people again. The stress of this only added to the hair loss problem so it was a vicious circle.

I started to be very gentle with my hair and careful with my diet. I have now found a hairdresser who works with me and understands the thinness of my hair and works around it. I am much more confident now about trying new styles and occasional colouring my hair. Using Nutrigro® Hair System made a marked improvement. I am less stressed most of the time now too and I think this has helped.

Male Pattern Baldness?

Case Study –Paul

Since the mid 30's my hair has been thinning on the top. I was more aware of it and felt self-conscious. I have been using Nutrigro® Hair System and have been very impressed, as my hair is definitely looking thicker, shinier and less dull looking.

Age?

Case Study-Helen

I am 63. My hair has been falling out and thinning at the front. My Doctor said that nothing could be done about it. I used a well-known tablet marketed for hair thinning but after 3 months I gave up on it, as it was not making any difference. After one month of using the Nutrigro® Hair System my hair has grown thicker at the front.

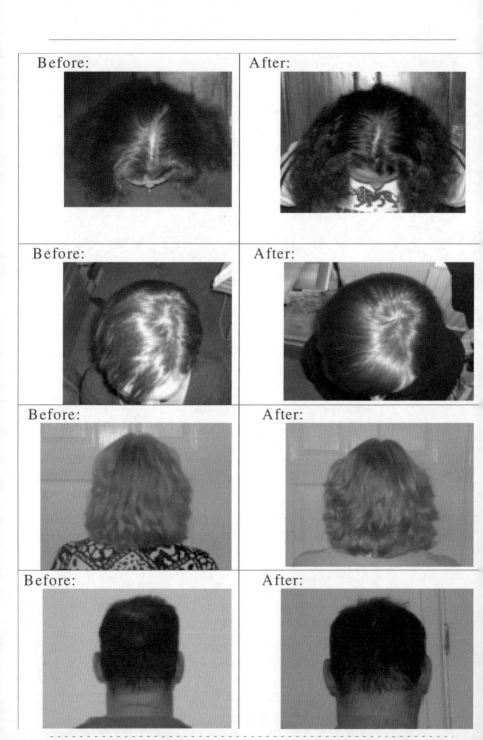

Before:

After:

Before:

After:

Before:

After:

Before:

After:

Chapter 14

Have you got the rare cause? - there is help

> *"If you were the only one with a problem –congrats you have just made history!"© Ravi Bhanot*

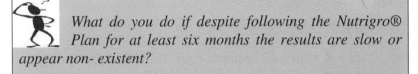
What do you do if despite following the Nutrigro®Plan for at least six months the results are slow or appear non- existent?

There is a possibility of heavy metal toxicity that needs looking at.

Metals such as Lead, Cadmium, Mercury, Iron, Aluminium and Copper are known to cause hair loss. Other elements such as Manganese, Chromium, Arsenic, and Titanium can also be involved. There is evidence that Lithium and Selenium can cause hair loss.

How do you know that you may have toxic metal poisoning? Blood tests do not usually show up heavy metals unless the person is suffering from a high level of poisoning. **The answer is to keep a look out on the fingernails.** Slow, long term exposure to the metals causes the nails to be abnormal.

Mercury affects the immune system by destroying T-cells. There are three kinds of cells that work in the immune system- B-cells, T-cells and T-8 cells. T-cells or 'helper' cells distinguish foreign cells to be attacked by B-cells, which surround and destroy these foreign cells. T-8 cells or 'suppressor' cells make sure that the B-cells do not attack normal tissues. When they do we see autoimmune conditions such as alopecia areata.

A research study in the early 1990's showed that around 50% of women with increased mercury in their body had hair loss. On removing mercury fillings around 65% saw hair coming back.

Be aware too that gold and amalgam fillings in the mouth can create electric currents in the mouth. These can affect your body's natural electromagnetic fields (1), which can result in poor health.

 What can you do to reduce mercury in the body?

Replace your mercury amalgam fillings for white ones. Only go to dentists who use a gumshield in your mouth when they do this to reduce exposure to mercury vapours when the filling is being removed. Do a detox and take *Nutrigro®* Hair capsules to get rid of remainders of mercury that have settled in the tissues.

Beware-some dentists are not even aware of mercury toxicity research and may discourage removal of mercury fillings!

To find a dentist who can help you with mercury-free dentistry visit www.amalgam.ukgo.com-The British Society for Mercury Free Dentistry or Mercury Free Association in USA (719-522-0566).

Toxic metals can cause both poor hair and nail growth and hair loss. Metal toxicity may produce white lines and horizontal ridges. Toxic metals or heavy metals are not easily removed from the body. They accumulate in the joints, bone, liver and other organs. They need to be removed, with advice from a Therapist, by taking specific supplements to neutralise them or chelate with them.

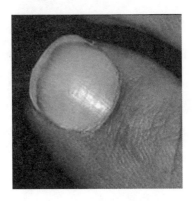

Where do you get heavy metal exposure? This can be from paint arts and crafts, electrical work, soldering, jewellery repair, pollution, cooking utensils, deodorants, and pesticides.

Chemical Toxicity

You may need to look at the chemical exposure in your environment. If you are on **medication check with your Pharmacist or Doctor** so see if your drugs are contributing to hair loss.

- **Pesticides, radiation treatment, chemotherapy, ionizing radiation such as UV and x-rays, radon, rancid oils, formaldehyde and benzene may all contribute.**

To test for toxic metal toxicity you can send us a small amount of hair for a hair-mineral analysis. Email me ravi@coolherbals.com for more information.

Chapter 15

Secrets from around the world for healthy hair

> *"World changing secrets are best kept open"*
> © –Ravi Bhanot

- To get extra protein into the hair use **6-8 drops of fresh lemon juice to an egg. Beat well and apply to your hair followed by washing with an herbal shampoo such as *Nutrigro*®.** We experimented with a mixture of egg and lemon juice for six months to get the smell and texture right but could we?! No chance! We even heated the eggs to make a paste out of them. I even went to India to see how this egg shampoo specialist made it! My conclusion is that the formulation is best used daily as described above.

- To soften hair you could **massage weekly with Rosemary Oil or Emu Oil.**

- **Mix yoghurt, lemon and mustard oil, and apply gently on the hair.** Wash your head after about half an hour and your hands - believe me you will need to! The theory of this is that yoghurt contains live lacto bacillus, a microorganism. This may counteract the effect of itchy scalps that have originated from yeast growths. Lemon would give the slightly acidic pH that is optimum for scalps. This may be a messy procedure though!

- **Use amla (100gm), shikaki (100gm), brahmi booti (root) (10gm), shilajit (1/2 gm), anaarchhilka (20gm) and bhringraj (10 gm) powders.** Soak them overnight in an iron utensil. Blend and make a paste of them. Apply the paste well into the scalp. Keep this paste on for 1-2 hours and wash off with warm water. This is an Indian formula, useful though hard work! I have trialled-using Amla and it does help thinning hair. I use it in my female hair food capsules formulation and *Nutrigro®* Female hair capsules. If you have any problems getting any of the above ingredients email me.

- **Prepare a hair tonic boiling dry pieces of Amla in coconut oil. Coconut oil is a hair moisturiser that enriches hair growth.** Soak two tablespoons of Fenugreek (methi) seeds overnight in water. The softened seeds are ground into a fine paste and applied over the scalp. This is left on the scalp for half an hour and then washed thoroughly. The Fenugreek improves blood circulation to the scalp and allows more nutrients to get to the hair. I have trialled-using Fenugreek with positive results. I use it in my *Nutrigro®* Female hair food capsules.

- **Rum Shampoo.** Mix two egg-yolks with two dessertspoonfuls of odourless linseed oil and two dessertspoonfuls of rum. Soak this into the hair and scalp. Keep this on for one hour and rinse off with warm water. This is especially good for dandruff and dry hair. If you have any rum left you can always drink it-it may at least make you forget your hair problem for a short while!

A preparation made from green cocoa beans, antioxidants and an Ayurvedic herb Indian pennywort has been used for women with variable results. This works by calming the immune system.

- **Scratching your nails.** Ayurvedic texts mention scratching nails of one hand horizontally across the nails of the other hand to promote stronger hair. Do one hand for a minute daily and then the other hand for one minute daily. I have a number of testimonials from clients who have found this to help reduce the rate of hair loss or bring back hair!

- **Massaging with essential oils.** Use 3 drops of rosemary oil, 3 drops lavender oil, 2 drops of cedarwood oil, 4 teaspoonfuls of grapeseed oil and 2.5ml of jojoba oil in Sesame Oil base. Alternatively you can buy Skinele Oil from select shops or from the Internet. This is a formulation that I devised using **a** blend of various oils such as sunflower oil, black mustard oil and sandalwood oil in sesame oil base - a balanced Vata, Pitta, Kapha oil suitable for all - visit www.ayurvedainstitute.org or www.ayurvedixpro.com for more information.

- **Massage hair and scalp with bulb onion juice to strengthen it**. The smell may be a bit of a put off though!

- **Extract of nettles** is applied to the scalp to prevent hair loss and stimulate hair growth.

Clever ways of making hair look thicker.

- **Colouring hair with a natural hair dye such as henna adds shine and vitality. This makes hair look healthier.**

- **A shorter cut makes hair look thicker and healthier.**

- Deeper richer colours of hair make hair look thicker.

- Women can use gentle self-grip rollers, which pump up the volume and make hair look thicker.

Chapter 16

How to arm yourself for the Specialist's door

• **If you are looking at hair restoration you will need to see a Doctor**. If the hair loss is caused by a reason other than genetics you would want to see a Dermatologist. If your hair loss is due to genetics then a general Doctor or Alternative Health Practitioner may do. For hairpieces you may need to visit a Trichologist, or a Hairdresser that specialises in this.

• **If you are looking for surgical intervention you would want to see a Doctor who specialises in this**. It is wise to do some initial reading before deciding on the choice of treatment. Books like this help, as does research on the Internet. If your hair loss is not due to genetics but perhaps due to dietary, disease or from medication then you could see an Alternative Health Professional or Trichologist.

• **If you would like Professional help visit a Trichologist, Doctor or an Alternative Health Practitioner.** A Trichologist specialises in hair and scalp problems. The title is not restricted and so you see various types of Trichologists-those that specialise in hair pieces to those who are hair stylists or those that work with Medical Doctors to be best able to help their clients. You can find a local one, in Britain from the following websites: www.hairscientists.org or from www.trichologists.org.uk.

These are some of the things to look out for:

Hair Loss Diagnosis

- Before **recommending treatment the Professional will conduct a scalp examination, overall physical and emotional health to determine the cause of hair loss**. Your medical history will be noted as well as your current medication.

- **Your hair will be assessed against standard hair loss charts such as Hamilton/Norwood for men and Ludwig for women**. The pattern of your hair loss is important as well as the character. Is there general thinness or is it receding or are there balding patches? How is the hair that is remaining? Are the hairs full sizes or are they fine and short? You will be asked if your close relatives –parents, grand parents, older brothers or sisters have had hair loss.

If it is thought to be hair loss other than male or female pattern baldness, the professional may seek the cause with other diagnostic measures.

Hair Pull

- **A hair pull is one such diagnostic procedure to assess the presence or absence of abnormalities in the hair growth cycle** About 25 to 50 hairs are removed from the scalp by this procedure. Only a few hairs are dislodged with each pull. If however more come out, this could be a possibility of an abnormal hair growth cycle. The ends of the pulled-out hairs can be examined under a microscope. This may show the condition of the hair shaft and the bulb (the end of the hair shaft extracted from the hair follicle).

There are various ways to hair pull- phototrichogram and hair window are two ways.

- **Phototrichogram**. This is where hairs are shaved in an area of the scalp. Consecutive photographs are taken over a period of 3 to 5 days to determine the hair growth pattern.

- **Hair window.** This is where hairs are shaved in an area of the scalp. The hair growth is evaluated over the next 3 to 30 days.

- It has to be said that **abnormalities of hair growth cycles is a relatively uncommon reason for hair loss. More usually the causes of hair abnormalities include thyroid hormone imbalance, nutritional deficiencies, side effects of certain drugs, anaemia and other systemic illnesses and psychological stress. A thyroid test or a Ferritin test could be ordered. There could be advice on changing your diet, your hair care or medication or there could be a referral to a Counsellor for example.**

- **Scalp Biopsy. A biopsy of the scalp can be done for additional information** to evaluate the mechanism of hair loss inside the hair follicle. This is usually not routinely done however.

Hair Analysis

- **A Hair analysis is a laboratory test that can be done to check if heavy metals are playing a part.**

Questions your Practitioner may ask:

Questionnaire on history of hair loss
When and how long have you had this problem?
What has been the pattern of hair loss?
Is hair coming out by the roots, or is it breaking along the hair?
Is increased hair loss or increased thinning more visible?
Are you taking any drugs?
Has the hair loss started in post- pregnancy or in menopause?

What has been your medical history like?
How is your thyroid gland functioning-has there been an increase in weight, lethargy?
Is there a family link to the hair loss?
Have you been using unusual hair care, hair cosmetics or hairstyle?
What is your diet like?

Differential diagnosis
If hair is coming from the roots-type of hair loss could be:
• Telogen effluvium
• Androgenic alopecia
• Alopecia areata
• Drug related

If hair is breaking type of hair loss could be:
• Tinea capitis
• Problems with structure of hair
• Breakage due to improper use of hair-care cosmetics
• Anagen stage of hair growth stopped

• If the cause of hair loss is one that cannot be reversed satisfactorily you could explore medication, surgery or hairpieces Some Trichologists specialise in hairpieces. Medication or surgery could be possible ways forward to discuss with your Doctor.

These are factors to consider before choosing a method of treatment for your hair loss or hair thinning:

Age: As you get older the harder it is to regrow hair.

How long has there been hair loss or hair thinning?
The longer there has been hair loss the more difficult it is to reverse the trend in Androgentic-type hair loss.

Have you recently started the menopause or given birth (for women)? This may indicate a hormonal imbalance.

What medications are you on?
Some medications as discussed earlier can affect your hair growth.

Is there a family history of diabetes, asthma, arthritis, vitiligo, anaemia, lupus or Addison's disease? These can all affect hair loss.

Has your hair become greyer at the same time as losing hair? Generally grey older hair is harder to regrow.

Are you serious about recognizing your problem, choosing the correct treatment and sticking to it? Once you recognize the cause – which could be diet, medication and/ or life style, you may be more motivated to stick to the plan of action of treatment.

If one treatment does not work are you prepared to try another treatment?
Sometimes you have to try different treatments - you may need to try different ones till one works for you. Having said this, bearing in mind the typical hair growth cycle, you will need to give any treatment about 3 months to work. Some medications have been tested for use for one year to see if they work- patience is a virtue!

Some treatments can be expensive-check the costs and probable length of treatment before commencing.

Are you willing to continue any successful treatment for a long term? With most treatments they work whilst you are taking or using the products involved. Some cause an increase in hair loss initially before positive benefits are seen.

The medications prescribed by Doctors

There are 5 types of treatments for the different causes of male and female hair loss.

DHT Inhibitors:

- As discussed before **too much DHT production causes an imbalance in the biology of the hair follicle resulting in the hair growth slowing down. Treatments that reduce or stop the production of DHT are getting to the root of the problem**

- **Super Oxide Dismutase Treatments or Immune System Treatments:**

When excess DHT is produced the scalp sometimes gets inflamed. Our bodies mistakenly assume that our hair follicles are foreign objects and they start attacking them. When the body sees the hair follicles as foreign objects it produces Super Oxides. To curtail the level of Super Oxides some treatments contain Super Oxide Dismutase treatments to lower the levels of Super Oxides.

- **Growth Stimulators:**
These do not address the cause of the problem but merely cosmetically promote hair growth.

- **Anti-Androgens:**
One of the main causes of hair loss is due to DHT binding to the Androgen receptors. DHT inhibitors reduce or stop the levels of DHT. Anti-Androgens stop the DHT binding to the Androgen receptors and in this way stop hair follicles from being damaged.

- **Anti-Inflammatory:**

As described **above when the immune system attacks hair follicles, as it assumes that they are foreign entities, the scalp becomes inflamed, flaky and itchy. These anti-inflammatories help with these symptoms.**

The common prescription medications available for hair loss are Finasteride, Minoxidil and a few varieties of lotions of Minoxidil with other drugs.

Finasteride is a DHT Inhibitor.

Finasteride (Propecia) was originally made to shrink prostate glands. In 1998 it was also approved at a lower dosage of 1mg as a treatment for hair loss. Finasteride as a 5mg strength tablet is used to treat prostate enlargement. **It blocks the enzyme 5 alpha reductase that converts Testosterone into DHT**, a form that enlarges the prostate gland. **Testosterone is also responsible for some genetically predisposed hair follicle cells to miniaturize.** This eventually leads to hair loss. By blocking the conversion of Testosterone from one form to another Finasteride helps stop hair loss. In some cases significant hair regrowth is also seen.

- A two-year study showed 83% of men taking Finasteride maintained hair at the top part of their heads (vertex area) compared to 28% of men taking a placebo. In the same study 17% of the men taking Finasteride still lost a significant amount of hair whereas 72% of the men taking the placebo also lost additional hair. After the first two years, results of the group taking Propecia continued to improve.

- There can be some possible side effects, although it must be emphasised that this is only seen in a small number of people. **Because of the nature of how it works, Finasteride is only recommended for men**. It can shrink the prostate gland in men susceptible to an enlarged prostate. Finasteride treatment may cause a loss of sex drive in 1-2% of patients as a result of reducing levels of DHT circulating in the blood. There is a risk of reducing the volume of ejaculate by up to 20% if the prostate gland is reduced in size although sperm activity appears to remain normal.

Minoxidil

- Minoxidil's hair stimulating properties were discovered when it was originally taken in trial patients as a treatment for high blood pressure. **It has been clinically proven to cause hair growth, particularly around the vertex of the scalp, although the precise mechanism of its working is unclear. It is thought to shorten the dormant (sleeping) resting phase of the hair follicle through the opening of potassium channels. Some think it works because it is a vasodilator - it makes blood vessels bigger around hair follicles and stimulates growth**. The results do however vary. In 1983 Dr. C. King showed two out of four people with alopecia areata had full recovery with a 3% solution but no one with total hair loss had any success (1) whereas Dr. Hinderson in 1984 reported a 80% success rate out of 53 patients, including one with complete hair loss (2). Results with Minoxidil show that hair count increases for the first 18-24 months before they stabilise. Encouragingly people using the medication over a longer period still had an increase in hair count after five years.

• **Some mild reddening and dryness of the scalp may be seen in some Minoxidil users due to the alcoholic nature of the lotion. A sebum removing shampoo such as the** *Nutrigro®* **hair shampoo can be used with Minoxidil**.

• Unlike Propecia, Minoxidil can be safely used for women in its 2% solution. Many women use and have reported improved effects with the use of the 5% solution, although the Manufacturers recommend that this stronger version should be used by men only.

• Since **Minoxidil's method of action does not involve DHT inhibition it can be used with other drugs such as inasteride or** *Nutrigro®* **Hair Food capsules, Serum or Shampoo or Conditioner.** When using the *Nutrigro®* Serum it is best to apply it at a different time to ensure maximum absorption.

• **Minoxidil can be combined with Tretinoin or Retinoic acid to promote hair growth.** The Journal of the American Academy of Dermatology cites several cases in which the use of Retinoic acid alone prompted striking hair growth. A 43 year old woman with androgenetic alopecia for over 20 years saw a 110% increase in hair count over a period of 18 months. Minoxidil With Retinoic acid combination showed a significant response in 66% of people, with 44% placed in the good response group and 22% in the moderate response group. The placebo people showed no significant hair growth response. As a Pharmacist I make and supply this formulation –it is not the first choice for most octors but may be worth trying if Minoxidil on its own has been unsatisfactory. If you are a Professional you may want to visit our website www.trichologysupplies.co.uk for more details on choices of medications.

- Retinoic acid reduces the chemical bonding between skin cells. **This causes hair that is in the Telogen (resting) phase to come out more readily** -bear in mind they would have come out anyway. It is thought that Retinoic acid increases the absorption of Minoxidil reaching the hair follicles. There is evidence that Retinoic acid itself helps hair growth.

- There are postulated to be two mechanisms by which Retinoic acid promotes hair growth in combination with Minoxidil. **Experimental evidence suggests that Retinoic acid 0.025% itself may play a significant role in hair growth** (1). It should be added that exposure to the sun should be kept to the minimum, as Retinoic acid decomposes with strong sunlight. Whilst using Retinoic acid, an initial mild irritation and redness of the skin frequently occurs.

- Tretinoin can be used with Minoxidil too. Results show that there is a **three-fold increase in the absorption of Minoxidil when used with Tretinoin**.

Ketoconazole, an anti-fungal, can also be used as a shampoo or with Minoxidil as it has been shown that it interacts with the androgen receptor.

Why aren't the results with these medications better than they are? I think it is because we need to take on a holistic approach to hair loss. Evidence is strongly suggesting that nutrition, hair care system, breathing technique, positive outlook, a proper method of shampoo and massage need to be considered too.

The sooner Hair Health Professionals (Doctors, Trichologists, and Dermatologists) realize and adopt a more holistic approach, the better the results would be for clients. Train yourselves on the techniques shown in this book (Nutrigro® Plan)- based on tried and tested ancient techniques- on teaching your clients nutrition, breathing techniques, life style changes and massage techniques- for a better future. We can change the trend of thinning hair and hair loss and not necessarily through drugs.

We look forward to the days when more Professionals such as Trichologists, Hairdressers, Pharmacists, Health Food shop operators and Doctors start educating their clients to adopt the right shampooing method, offer techniques like the Ayurvedic head massages and teach their clients some of the techniques described in this book. This would be a step towards taking the whole subject of hair thinning and hair loss more seriously.

I know some Professionals are going to say that they have never done this before so why start now and some will be say this is not their domain. Maybe. The world is crying for a new approach to keeping hair for longer. Why not learn new skills to make treatment holistic? Please see the following websites for more information: www.ayurvedainstitute.org, and www.coolherbals.com. If I can help you to make a difference to your clients contact me at ravi@coolherbals.com.

Chapter 17

Answers to burning questions

> *"To every Jack there is a Jill, to every problem a solution"* -
> ©*Ravi Bhanot*

Does stress make you lose hair?

• **Does stress cause hair loss or does the cause of hair loss cause stress?** There are conflicting medical reports of whether stress makes you lose hair. What complicates matters is that hair loss due to stress is delayed by a few weeks to a few months- so was it stress that caused hair loss? **Generally speaking it is not stress, but the ability to deal with stress that makes the difference in people losing hair due to stress.**

Does wearing a cap or hat cause hair loss?

• **Research shows that people with poor circulation due to tight caps or hats do not necessarily appear to be more likely to suffer from alopecia.** It is only in a very small minority of people that this is seen. This may be due to impairment of blood flow in the scalp. The advice is alopecia sufferers should take caution in wearing tight caps and hats.

Does dirty or unkempt hair damage hair and make it fall out?

• There is no evidence for this.

Does frequent shampooing cause hair loss?

- Authorities recommend that care should be taken with fragile and thinning hair. Using natural, gentle, non-harsh chemical shampoos is better than harsh chemical shampoos. Any tangles of hair should be carefully separated making sure you are not pulling the hair. **It is not the frequency you wash your hair that counts, but what shampoo and conditioner you use.**

Do perms, colours and other cosmetic treatments cause permanent hair loss?

- **Some hair treatments can damage the hair and lead to alopecia-but the vast majority do not.** So if you are experiencing hair loss after using perms or colourants then avoid them.

Do women lose more hair than men?

- **Not necessarily.**

Does shaving the head make the hair grow back thicker?

- **Not true -** in fact, if you are suffering from Androgenetic Alopecia, this will actually just quicken your hair loss.

Does standing on one's head cause increased circulation and thereby stimulate hair growth?

- I am afraid there is no evidence to support for this.

Does dandruff cause permanent hair loss?

Do you lose more hair at certain times of the year?

- **Yes some do,** according to a set of scientists. Circannual rhythms (physiological variations that occur in the same period of the year) can be described as a change in the level of hormones secreted by your body. Scientists believe that these fluctuations explain many pathologies (the scientific study of the nature of disease and its causes) such as male pattern baldness. A study called the "Tromsø study" screened all inhabitants aged 25 years or older living in Tromsø (Norway) for their Testosterone blood levels over a period of time.

The study showed that Testosterone reaches two peaks during the year, one in February-March and the other one in November-December (Figure 1). **As can be seen from the graph below the biggest peak is in Autumn.**

Figure 1 – Shows Total Testosterone (Total-T) and free Testosterone (Free-T) levels during a 12-month period.

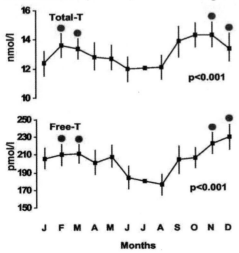

- It has also been observed by some scientists that more hair is lost in Spring and in Autumn. **This coincides with the Tromsø study that shows a seasonal variation (of about 30% by season) of total and free testosterone** (Figure 2).

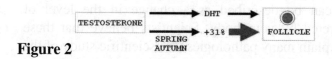

Figure 2

So why does more hair fall out in these seasons? **It is postulated that Spring and Autumn both see a sudden change in climate-both temperature and amount of daylight.** These sudden variations in the factors may be stressing the body The body responds by releasing the hormone, Testosterone. Higher Testosterone blood levels means more DHT in the scalp and consequently less hair on your scalp. (You may recall from earlier that DHT attacks hair follicles.)

Chapter 18

What is around the corner to help your hair?

"Future is based on experience, experience is based on failures and failures are based on experimentation...I wonder which experiments we should be working on."
© Ravi Bhanot

- Future treatments for hair loss will include **novel treatments such as hair follicle cloning and gene therapy. Cosmetic treatments may be products that make hair look fuller.**

- The **present drugs for hair loss have limited effectiveness.** They need to be taken on continuously and they have a limited visual impact on some people. The drugs are not cheap either.

- A new drug, **Dutasteride, is similar to Finasteride in its action but it has a more dramatic effect** in reducing the amount of Testosterone being converted to Dihydrotestosterone (DHT), in the blood. DHT causes a reduction in hair growth in those people who are genetically affected and who are also sensitive to DHT. Women too will benefit from Dutasteride because it works on type I alpha-reductase enzyme too-the enzyme that promotes quicker conversion of Testosterone to DHT. There are two types of 5-alpha-reducatase that convert Testosterone to DHT. Whereas Propecia only works on type II, Dutasteride works on both. Propecia causes up to 70% reduction decrease in DHT in male blood, Dutasteride causes around 90%.

- **More topical lotions, shampoos and conditioners will be available in the future that target hair loss causing cells. These would help in reducing side effects. This is the thinking behind** *Nutrigro®* **hair products.**

- **Drugs will also be made to keep hair longer in the Anagen or growth phase of the hair cycle** and those that override the signal for hair to leave the hair growth phase. There will also be drugs for treating diseases that cause hair loss.

- Genetics will also give us answers to hair loss and regrowth. **Gene therapy is changing the genes of existing cells causing a change in cell function**. This involves finding out the inherited medical condition with respect to the DNA at its molecular level and then fixing the error or errors. This therapy is still being investigated.

In essence the hair follicles that are DHT-sensitive cells need to be made DHT-resistant so that hairs continue growing on a long-term basis. However we do not know all the genes involved in the cycle of hair growth or those involved for inherited hair loss.

In 1998 **Dr Angelo Christiano identified a single gene, called** *hairless*, **causing a rare type of inherited baldness called generalised atrichia**(1). American scientists and scientists in Pakistan studied a family whose members frequently had alopecia universalis (no scalp or body hair growth after birth). Scientists wondered whether it might be that the human version of a mouse gene, when mutated, resulted in hairless rodents. Using the DNA sequence of the mouse gene, they found the human version in the chromosomal region they had targeted. Researchers think that the gene stores a mutation in family members afflicted with alopecia universalis.

The scientists hope that their discovery will lead to the identification of more genes involved in human hair growth. Such research may result in new treatments to slow or reverse hair loss. More time is needed for research. Genes need to be identified and the changing of DNA codes needs working out.

The research however shows that it is possible to genetically modify hair follicles. The process of removing a small number of follicle cells, introducing new genetic material to them and then re-implanting the engineered cells into an organism may work. This shows the possible ability to transfer genetic information from one organism and that the hair shaft could be modified.

- **Cloning is another exciting way forward.** Cloning is a technique of reproducing cells, organs or organisms from a single cell compared to reproduction where there is mixing of DNA from two parents. Cloning results in the offspring having the same DNA blueprint as the parent. This could be of use where the parent's DNA has resistance to DHT. The technique needs more time to be perfected and then at an affordable price.

> *There is still hope...just keep your hair on!*

Chapter 19

Summary: Bring it back-hair and all

"What the mind sees first the eye sees second" -
© Ravi Bhanot

Keep the following summary of the Plan to stick somewhere you will see everyday…. make it second nature.

1. **Follow the** *Nutrigro®* **Diet**- keeping your food 70% alkaline and emphasise on Pitta pacifying foods-see Appendix1.
2. **Supplement your diet with Vitamins and Minerals** that give "food" to the hair-two capsules daily of the *Nutrigro®* Male or Female Hair Food capsules. You may need the *Nutrigro®* Hair Food Plus capsules if you have post pregnancy, menopausal or hormone imbalanced hair loss or hair thinning.
3. **Drink 2-2.5 litres of water if you are a man or 1.5 litres if you are a woman**. This will flush away toxins and bring in nourishment to the cells.
4. **Do the Scalp and Ayurvedic Head massage daily.**
5. **Exercise at least three times a week -** 20 minutes of aerobic exercises. **Vigorously brush your tongue** first thing every morning after brushing your teeth until you feel you are about to bring something up.
6. **Use the right hair care products** for hair that is thinning or being lost. Use the *Nutrigro®* Hair Serum, Shampoo and Conditioner. Use the Serum daily, the Shampoo at least twice a week and the Conditioner once a week.
7. **Visualize every night** before going to sleep that you are retaining the hair you have, that it is getting healthier, thicker and stronger. You are losing less hair and hair is regrowing. Have this as a large coloured picture that you can feel, touch and see. Be grateful for the hair you have. Have a positive mind. Affirm to yourself that you are doing the best you could be doing for your hair, naturally. Have a photo of the hair you would like to have stuck somewhere you see it everyday-on

would like to have stuck somewhere you see it everyday - on your cupboard door or on your computer for example. Leave the rest to the Universe. Use methods to reduce stress. Remember: How you communicate with yourself is the most important communication.

8. **Breathe right.** Exercise 1: Use the 4-2-8 method. Breathe in through one nostril whilst the other is closed, with the stomach expanding out-count to 4, hold for 2 with both nostrils closed and breathe out through the other nostril whilst the other is closed forcing the stomach to contract. Count to 4.

Exercise 2: **Force air out through both nostrils with the stomach going in as you do so.** Do this quickly at a rate of about one every 2 seconds.

Repeat both above times 10, at least once a day in the morning and ideally at night too.

Appendix 1 - *Nutrigo* Diet Chart

These are foods to concentrate on to rebalance the pitta dosha.

Grains: Rice, wheat, barley, oats, all cooked until tender

Vegetables: Asparagus, tender and bitter greens, carrots, fennel peas, green beans, artichoke, parsnips, okra, celery, brussels sprouts, broccoli, cauliflower, beets, sweet potatoes, small quantities of raw lettuce, carrots or cucumber

Fruits: Avocado, pineapple, peaches, plums, grapes, mangoes, melons, pears, pomegranates, cherries, all kinds of berries, apples, coconut, dates, fresh and dried figs, raisins (soaked), all ripe and sweet

Lentils: Mung beans, mung dhal, red or brown lentils, black beans

Dairy: Whole milk, cream, butter, fresh yogurt (cooked into foods), lassi, cottage cheese

Oils: Olive oil, walnut oil

Herbs: Parsley, fresh basil, fresh fennel, fresh mint

Nuts and Seeds: Almonds (soaked and blanched), sunflower seeds, pumpkin seeds

Spices: Turmeric, cumin, cardamom, coriander, fennel, small quantities of black pepper, mint, saffron, dill

Other: Rice milk, soymilk, and tofu in moderation (diced small and cooked with spices)

Typical *Nutrigro®* Menus

Breakfast:
Shredded Wheat/ Rice Cereal/ Oatmeal/ Muffin/ French toast/ Pancakes/ Waffles/ Whole wheat toast/ Sweet fruit in season, Pear, Apple, Green Smoothies/ Milk/ Tea/ Soy Milk/ Coconut Milk/ Herb Tea (Chamomile, Mint, Lemon Grass, Chrysanthemum)

Lunch:
Large tossed salad/ Basmati Rice/ Whole wheat tortilla or bread/ Chapattis/ Broccoli or Cauliflower soup/ egg or asparagus salad/ Cottage cheese/ Baked Potato/ Rice cakes/ Coleslaw
-See other suitable foods in chart

Dinner:
Red kidney beans/ Rice/ Potatoes/ Corn on the cob/ Salads/ Soups/ Chinese Tofu Stir Fry/ Chinese vegetables/ Plain Rice
-See other suitable foods in chart

Dessert:
Rice pudding/ Puddings/ Tapioca/ Pumpkin pie

Fruits	Suitable	Unsuitable
Apples (cooked)	✔	
Apples (raw, sour)		✖
Apples (raw, sweet)	✔	
Apple sauce	✔	
Apricots (sour)		✖
Apricots (sweet)	✔	
Avocado	✔	
Bananas		✖
Berries (sour)		✖
Berries (sweet)	✔	
Cherries		✖
Coconut	✔	
Cranberries		✖
Dates (dry)	✔	
Dates (fresh)	✔	
Figs (dry)	✔	
Figs (fresh)	✔	
Grapefruit		✖
Grapes (green)		✖
Grapes (red)	✔	
Kiwi		✖
Lemons		✖

Limes	✓	
Mangoes (green)		✗
Mangoes (ripe)	✓	
Melons	✓	
Oranges (sour)		✗
Oranges (sweet)	✓	
Papaya		✗
Peaches		✗
Pears	✓	
Pineapple (sour)		✗
Pineapple (sweet)	✓	
Plums (sour)		✗
Plums (sweet)	✓	
Pomegranates	✓	
Prunes (dry)	✓	
Prunes (soaked)	✓	
Raisins (dry)	✓	
Raisins (soaked)	✓	
Rhubarb		✗
Strawberries		✗
Tamarind		✗
Watermelon	✓	

SWEETNERS	PITTA
Barley Malt	✔
Fructose	✔
Honey	✖
White Sugar	✔
Rice syrup	✔

SPICES	PITTA
Ajwan	✖
All spices	✖
Almond extract	✖

NUTS	PITTA
Almonds (with skins)	✖
Almonds (soaked and peeled)	✔
Black Walnuts	✖
Brazil Nuts	✖
Cashews	✖
Charole	✔
Coconut	✔
Walnuts	✖
Hazelnuts	✖
Peanuts	✖

Anise		✖
Asafoetida (hing)		✖
Basil (dry)		✖
Basil (fresh)	✔	
Bay leaf		✖
Black pepper	✔	
Caraway		✖
Cardamom	✔	
Cayenne		✖
Cinnamon	✔	
Cloves		✖
Coriander	✔	
Cumin	✔	
Dill	✔	
Fennel	✔	
Fenugreek		✖
Garlic		✖
Ginger (dry)		✖
Ginger (fresh)	✔	
Mint	✔	
Mustard seeds		✖
Neem leaves	✔	
Nutmeg		✖
Orange peel	✔	
Oregano		✖
Paprika		✖
Parsley	✔	

Peppermint	✓
Pippali	✗
Poppy Seeds	✗
Rosemary	✗
Saffron	✓
Sage	✗
Salt	✗
Savoury	✗
Spearmint	✓
Thyme	✗
Turmeric	✓
Vanilla	✓

MEAT, FISH & POULTRY	**PITTA**
Beef	✗
Chicken (white)	✓
Duck	✗
Eggs (white and yolk)	✗
Eggs (white only)	✓
Fish (freshwater)	✓
Fish (sea)	✗
Lamb	✗
Pork	✗
Salmon	✗
Sardines	✗
Seafood	✗

Shrimp	✓	
Tuna		✗
Turkey (white)	✓	

DAIRY	PITTA	
Butter (salted)		✗
Butter (unsalted)	✓	
Buttermilk		✗
Cheese (hard)		✗
Cheese (soft)	✓	
Cottage cheese	✓	
Cow's milk	✓	
Ghee	✓	
Goat's cheese	✓	
Goat's milk	✓	
Ice Cream	✓	
Sour Cream		✗
Yoghurt (plain, frozen or with fruit)		✗
Yoghurt (diluted and spiced)	✓	

LEGUMES	PITTA
Black beans	✓
Black eyed peas	✓
Chick peas (garbanzos)	✓
Kidney beans	✓
Lentils (brown)	✓
Lentils (red)	✓
Lima Beans	✗
Miso	✗
Mung beans	✓
Mung dal (lentils)	✓
Navy beans	✓
Peas (dried)	✓
Soy beans	✓
Soy Cheese	✓
Soy Flour	✓
Soy milk	✓
Soy powder	✓
Soy sauce	✗
Soy sausages	✗
Split peas	✓
Tofu (cold)	✓
Tofu (hot)	✓
Tur dal (lentils)	✗
Urad dal (lentils)	✗

		PITTA
White beans	✔	

SEEDS

		PITTA
	✔	
Popcorn (no salt, butter)	✔	
Psyllium	✔	
Pumpkin	✔	
Sesame		✖
Sunflower	✔	
Flax		✖

GRAINS

		PITTA
Amaranth	✔	
Barley	✔	
Bread (with yeast)		✖
Buckwheat		✖
Cereals (cold, dry or puffed)	✔ (dry only)	
Corn		✖
Couscous	✔	
Crackers	✔	
Millet		✖

Food		
Muesli		✗
Oat bran	✓	
Oats (dry)		✗
Oats (cooked)	✓	
Pancakes	✓	
Pasta	✓	
Rice (brown, white)		✗ (brown only)
Rice (Basmati, wild)	✓	
Rice cakes	✓	
Rye		✗
Spelt	✓	
Sprouted wheat beat (essence)	✓	
Tapioca	✓	
Wheat	✓	
Wheat bran	✓	

FOOD SUPPLEMENTS	PITTA	
Amino acids	✓	
Barley green		✗
Bee Pollen	✓	
Brewers yeast		✗
Royal jelly	✓	

For more information visit www.coolherbals.com

	PITTA	
Spirulina	✓	
Vitamin A, B, B12, C, D, E	✓	

MINERALS   PITTA

	PITTA	
Calcium	✓	
Copper	✓	
Iron	✓	
Magnesium	✓	
Zinc	✓	

VEGETABLES   PITTA

	PITTA	
Artichoke	✓	
Asparagus	✓	
Beet greens		✗
Beets (raw)		✗
Beets (cooked)	✓	
Bitter melon	✓	
Broccoli	✓	
Brussels sprouts	✓	
Burdock root		✗
Cabbage (cooked)	✓	
Cabbage (raw)	✓	
Carrots (raw)		✗

Carrots (cooked)	✔	
Cauliflower (cooked)	✔	
Cauliflower (raw)	✔	
Celery	✔	
Corn		✖
Cucumber	✔	
Radish		✖
Dandelion greens	✔	
Eggplant		✖
Fennel (Anise)	✔	
Garlic		✖
Green beans	✔	
Green chillies		✖
Horseradish		✖
Kale	✔	
Leafy greens	✔	
Leeks (cooked)	✔	
Leeks (raw)		✖
Lettuce	✔	
Mushrooms	✔	
Mustard Greens		✖
Okra	✔	
Olives (black)	✔	
Olives (green)		✖
Onions (raw)		✖

Onions (cooked)	✓	
Parsley	✓	
Parsnips	✓	
Peas (raw)	✓	
Peas (cooked)	✓	
Peppers (sweet)	✓	
Peppers (hot)		✗
Potatoes (white)	✓	
Prickly pear (fruit)		✗
Prickly pear (leaves)	✓	
Pumpkin	✓	
Radish (raw)		✗
Radish (cooked)	✓	
Spaghetti	✓	
Spinach (cooked)	✓	
Spinach (raw)		✗
Sprouts	✓	
Sweet potato	✓	
Tomatoes (cooked)		✗
Tomatoes (raw)		✗
Turnip greens		✗
Turnips		✗
Watercress	✓	
Wheat grass sprouts	✓	
Zucchini	✓	

CONDIMENTS

PITTA

Condiment	Pitta
Black pepper	✓
Chilli pepper	✓
Chocolate	✗
Chutney, mango (sweet)	✓
Chutney, mango (spicy)	✗
Coriander leaves	✓
Horseradish	✗
Kelp	✗
Ketchup	✗
Lemon	✗
Lime	✓
Lime pickle	✗
Mango pickle	✗
Mayonnaise	✗
Mustard	✗
Pickles	✗
Salt	✗
Scallions	✗
Seaweed	✓
Soy sauce	✗
Sprouts	✓
Vinegar	✗

Beverages	PITTA	
Apple Juice	✔	
Alcohol (beer)	✔	
Alcohol (hard)		✖
Alcohol (wine)		✖
Almond milk	✔	
Aloe Vera juice	✔	
Apple cider		✖
Apricot juice	✔	
Berry juice	✔	
Black tea	✔	
Caffeinated beverages		✖
Carbonated drinks		✖
Carob	✔	
Carrot juice		✖
Chai (hot spiced milk)	✔	
Cherry juice		✖
Chocolate milk		✖
Coffee		✖
Cold dairy drinks	✔	
Cranberry juice		✖
Grain 'coffee'	✔	
Grape juice	✔	
Grapefruit juice		✖
Iced tea		✖

Icy cold drinks	✗
Lemonade	✗
Mango juice	✓
Mixed veg. juice	✓
Orange juice	✗
Papaya juice	✗
Peach nectar	✓
Pear juice	✓
Pineapple juice	✗
Pomegranate juice	✓
Prune juice	✓
Rice milk	✓
Soy milk (cold)	✓
Soy milk (hot & well-spiced)	✗
Sour juices	✗
Tomato juice	✗
V-8 juice	✗

Herb Teas	Pitta	
Ajwan		✗
Alfalfa	✓	
Bancha	✓	
Barley	✓	
Basil		✗

Blackberry	✓
Borage	✓
Burdock	✓
Catnip	✓
Chamomile	✓
Chicory	✓
Chrysanthemum	✓
Cinnamon	✗
Clove	✗
Comfrey	✓
Dandelion	✓
Elderflower	✓
Eucalyptus	✗
Fennel	✓
Fenugreek	✓
Ginger	✓
Ginseng	✗
Hawthorn	✗
Hibiscus	✓
Hops	✓
Jasmine	✓
Juniper berry	✗
Lavender	✓
Lemon balm	✓
Lemon grass	✓

		Pitta
Liquorice	✓	
Marshmallow	✓	
Nettle	✓	
Orange peel	✓	
Passion flower	✓	
Pennyroyal		✗
Peppermint	✓	
Raspberry	✓	
Red clover	✓	
Rosehip		✗
Saffron	✓	
Sage		✗
Spearmint	✓	
Strawberry	✓	
Violet	✓	
Wintergreen	✓	
Yarrow	✓	
Oils		**Pitta**
Almond		✗
Apricot		✗
Avocado	✓ (external use only)	
Coconut	✓ (external use only)	
Corn		✗

Flax Seed	☑
Ghee	☑
Olive	☑
Primrose	☑
Safflower	✖
Sesame	✖
Soy	☑
Sunflower	☑
Walnut	☑

References

Chapter 1
(1) Hairdressing the Foundations, Green and Paladino's: published by Thompson Learning ISBN 0-333-69338-8
(2) Drs Arthur Rook and Rodney Dawber, Diseases of the Hair and the Scalp (Blackwell Scientific, 1982)

Chapter 2
(1) Hamilton, JB Male hormone stimulation is a prerequisite and an incitant in common baldness. Am J Anat, 1942. 71, 451–480
(2) JA Ellis, M Stebbing, SB Harrap - Journal of Investigative Dermatology, 1998 - Blackwell Synergy
(3) Dr A.J.M Penders, 'Alopecia Areata and Atophy', Dermatologica (1968) 136:395

Chapter 3
(1) Dr Hoffman, H.G.Meiers and A.Hubbes, Deutsche Medizinische Wochenshrift (1974),99:2151-1
(2) Conrad F, Paus R J Dtsch Dermatol Ges. 2004 Jun; 2(6): 412-23
(3) Tanriverdi N, Duru C, Saray Y, Akcali C Int J Dermatol. 2004 May; 43(5) 352-6

Chapter 4
(1) Nematian J, Ravaghi M, Gholamrezanezhad A, Nematian E. Am J Clin Dermatol. 2006; 7(4): 263-6
(2) Drs S.Muller and R.K.Winkelmann, 'Alopecia Areata', Archives of Dermatology (1963) 88:290
(3)   R.Finke Med Monatsschr Pharm 2001 May; 24(5): 147-53.

Chapter 5
(1)   Hort W, Nilles M, Mayser P. Hautarzt. 2006 Jul; 57(7): 633-43; quiz 644-5

Chapter 6
(1)   The Borneo Post - NH/16/16
(2)   N Prager, K Bickett, N French, G Marcovici - Journal of Alternative and Complementary Medicine, 2002
(3)   Walsh, DS, Dunn, CL, James, WD Improvement in androgenetic alopecia (stage V) using topical minoxidil in a retinoid vehicle and oral finasteride. Arch Dermatol, 1995. 134, 1373–1375
(4)   Sawaya, ME & Price, J Invest Dermatol, 1997. 109, 296–30
(5)   Cosmetic, Toiletry, and Fragrance Association (CTFA)-SLS and eye

Chapter 9
(1)   Dr Sears, *The Zone*- sugar levels
(2)   A.Johnson, J.Tilly, J.Levorse, Biology of Reproduction 44,338-344 (1991)- arachidonic acid and testosterone
(3)   Young Robert-*pH Miracle Living*
(4)   Anthony Robbins- *Unleash the Power Within*
(5)   Dr.M.Morter-*An apple a Day 1996*
(6)   Barnard ND, Scialli AR, Hurlock D, Bertron P., Obstet Gynecol.2000 Feb; 95(2): 245-50
(7)   Traditional Indian medicine in dermatology. Clinics in Dermatology, Volume 17, Issue 1, Pages 41-47 H. Routh
(8)   J Nutr. 2005 Mar; 135(3): 584-91. -Soya and lowering DHT
(9)   Starka L, Hill M, Polacek V. -Hormonal Profile in men with premature androgenic alopecia [Article in Czech] Endokrinologicky ustav a IPVZ, Praha, Czech Republic.

Chapter 10
(1)   John Gray, *Men are from Mars Women are from Venus*

Chapter 11
(1)   Melanie Sachs, *Ayurvedic Beauty Care*

Chapter 12
(1) Swami Ram Dev, www.swamiramdevyoga.com
(2) Shri Shri Ravi Shankar-Teachers' Manual AOL-level www.artofliving.org and www.breathing.com

Chapter 14
(1) Lynne McTaggart, The WDDTY Dental Handbook

Chapter 16
(1) Drs C.M.King and el. British Medical Journal (1983), 287:1380
(2) Dr C.Hinderson and el British Medical Journal (1984), 288:1087
(3) Bazzano et al Contact Dermatitis 3:55-56, 1977
(4) Science, January 30,1998, Vol.279, No.5351

Chapter 18
Science, January 30,1998, Vol.279, No.5351-Pakistani total